Praise for *When There Is No Cure*

"I wanted to cry just reading the table of contents. The author gets it! He understands the lonely path of those of us with chronic illness."
—*Elizabeth, a patient with lupus*

"This is a book that I wholeheartedly recommend for fellow sufferers of a chronic disease. It takes the reader on a journey that covers many of the concerns a person with a chronic disease has—such as how you can handle your illness, how to interact with doctors, how to handle other people's responses to your illness, and how others can help. I will use this as a guide in my journey with my chronic disease."

—*Lisa, a patient with dermatomyositis*

"You can feel the pain of his maladies and yet the author's powerful commitment to not allow it to affect the responsibilities of a father, a husband, or an educator. Most of all, I was moved by his heart in honestly sharing the journey that it might offer encouragement to those who find themselves similarly afflicted when there is no cure. This book should be required reading by every medical student."

—*Edward Langston, MD, family physician (retired)*
and former chairman of the Board of Trustees
for the American Medical Association

"This book touched my heart. It is filled with practical advice and hope for patients and healthcare providers. Very pertinent and encompassing, it is filled with pearls of wisdom. This book should be on the reading list of all who care for, live with, or know individuals with chronic suffering. His journey and acquired wisdom are a reminder that people can thrive despite a chronic disorder and that indeed 'life is more than good health.'"

—*Charles E. Sanders, Jr., MD, FACP, FACR,*
rheumatologist and former vice president of medical
education and research, Mount Carmel Health System

D0619804

When There Is No Cure

How to Thrive While Living with the
Pain and Suffering of Chronic Illness

Craig K. Svensson, PharmD, PhD

Important Note

This book provides general guidance for living with chronic illness. It is not intended to replace or subvert recommendations from a qualified healthcare provider nor discourage patients from seeking and following medical care. Healthcare decisions should be made in a collaborative manner between you and your healthcare provider. The author is not endorsing specific treatment plans and holds no liability for decisions patients make based on this book.

Patient names and minor details have been changed to protect their privacy.

When There Is No Cure: How to Thrive While Living with the Pain and Suffering of Chronic Illness

Cover design by: Cathi Stevenson, Book Cover Express

Paperback ISBN: 978-1-7327069-0-3
e-book ISBN: 978-1-7327069-1-0

Library of Congress Control Number: 2018914456

Consilium Publishing
West Lafayette, IN

In memory of my mother, Teresa Svensson, whose example of living with chronic illness taught me many valuable lessons.

Table of Contents

Introduction

A trio of pathological enemies work daily to disturb any sense of normalcy in my life. Pain rarely allows me to sleep more than two hours at a time. I have been reduced to a passive observer as my wife lifts or moves something heavy to prevent me from experiencing more intense back pain. My persistent standing when others are seated has stimulated remarkable comments—at times humorous, though more often rude or thoughtless. I could not count the many vacation options we have rejected over the years because they would require far more sitting than I could tolerate.

On too many occasions, I missed important events for our children because I was stuck in the bathroom with a flare of a chronic intestinal ailment. Responding to a dinner invitation at the home of others usually results in an embarrassing conversation for me or my wife. We must either provide them with a list of food ingredients to avoid or risk having me buckled over with intense abdominal pain shortly after dinner and then quickly checking out their indoor plumbing. Either way, people understandably often regret extending an invitation.

Rounding out the trifecta of ailments, several of my body parts emit a persistent burning pain or tingling. Standing is best for my back, but the bottom of one foot feels like it has a bad sunburn, while the other feels like it is being pricked by a thousand little pinheads. Do I stand or sit? Which hurts worse at the moment? Sometimes all three diseases conspire with one another to launch a simultaneous assault on my plans for the day. On other occasions, they take turns increasing the discomfort in my life. While these chronic conditions could overtake my life, I am not willing to surrender to their rule.

I am just one of millions who live with chronic medical conditions bearing ominous labels like systemic lupus erythematosus, fibromyalgia, multiple sclerosis, rheumatoid arthritis, and ulcerative colitis—just to name a few. There is no cure for what ails us. Pain and persistent suffering are expected parts of our future. Often the degree of both is certain to worsen as the years progress. Our illnesses are commonly invisible. The grimace with certain movements or the avoidance of other activities may be the only outward sign something is amiss with our bodies. Nevertheless, underneath the façade is a daily challenge to press on despite the discomfort. This is a well-worn path for me, and I have written this book to help others on a similar road.

The suffering brought about by our chronic illnesses can lead to dramatic changes in our lives. Activities that once brought us joy may no longer be possible.

Simple movements long taken for granted are now painful or exhausting. Body parts we have never given much thought to begin to scream for attention. The future, once so promising, seems rather bleak. Hope crashed into the hard rock of reality when the doctor said, "There's nothing more we can do."

You can thrive in the face of suffering brought on by chronic illness. You can know joy when parts of your body constantly rebel against their normal function. You can restore a sense of balance when illness has overturned the priorities and plans once carefully laid. But how do you do so?

I have been on a nearly thirty-five-year journey accumulating several incurable ailments. Each additional malady has brought with it a host of unwanted alterations in how I live life. But this experience has also taught me that, yes, those of us living with chronic conditions can thrive in the face of our long-term suffering. Sadly, I have seen many who do not. Often their failure to live well is not due to the incurable ailment itself but rather to their response to this unwanted companion bringing havoc to their body. We cannot control the arrival of pathological invaders into our lives. What you can control is your response to these uninvited diseases. Your response is what will determine your ability to thrive in the face of a life-altering ailment.

In my professional and personal travels across the country, I visited many bookstores and posed a simple question to the booksellers: "What book would you recommend to someone diagnosed with an incurable, but not fatal, illness?" The frequent response was a perplexed look, sometimes accompanied by scratching the head or chin. At best, they directed me to books focused on living a healthy lifestyle—often through a diet plan of unproven value. A few pointed to books focused on a very specific disease. These invariably dealt with an unconventional and poorly supported approach to treatment. But all the booksellers were at a loss for a book that addresses the many issues faced by those of us living with incurable ailments that lead to many years of an altered lifestyle, such as:

- How do we get physicians to take our health complaints seriously?

- Where do we turn when doctors acknowledge our ailment with upturned hands and confess they don't know how to help?

- How do we deal with the overwhelming sense of loss upon receiving an untreatable diagnosis—one sure to produce profound changes in our life?

- How do we address those whose reaction to our ailment increases our suffering?

- Can we live well with inescapable pain?

- How do we avoid living in a state of fear when facing an uncertain prognosis?

- Should we try to keep our disease
  a secret from others?

- How do we choose between treatment
  options when each could cause harm?

- How do we tell if new symptoms are from our
  chronic disease or signs of some new ailment?

- How do we live with regret when an
  ailment is a result of choices we made?

- How can those who love us help?

I address these questions in the chapters ahead.

What qualifies me to write a book on living with the chronic suffering an incurable ailment brings? I trained as a clinical pharmacist, learning to manage drug therapy for patients with acute and chronic disease. Later, I earned a second doctorate with a focus on pharmaceutical research. My own research career focused on adverse reactions from drugs. Throughout my professional career, I have educated future nurses, pharmacists, physicians, and physician assistants on the fundamental principles of drug therapy—how drugs act in the body, how to select which drugs to use for what conditions, and how to deal with side effects and adverse reactions.

In addition to my formal training and clinical experience, education relevant to this book came from being a patient myself. In the mid-1980s, I developed a rare form of colitis for which there were, and remain, no proven treatments. In 1997, I experienced a back injury leaving me with unremitting pain that remains to this day—though less intense than the first decade. Then, in 2005, symptoms of multiple sclerosis (MS) began to emerge. Repeated relapses have left me with a variety of persistent symptoms not responsive to treatment.

My personal experience has helped me better understand the experience voiced by others. I knew of people who grumbled about the difficulty of getting healthcare providers to take their complaints seriously. I sensed their frustration and felt sorry for them. But it was not until I walked the same road and experienced these frustrations that I actually *understood* what they were saying. I heard patients express a sense of helplessness in living with the diagnosis of an incurable ailment. After experiencing and needing to deal with those feelings through my own diagnoses, my eyes have opened in a manner only experience can accomplish.

Having lived most of my adult life on a journey through an unexplainable series of such ailments, I now better identify with the troubled existence of many of my fellow travelers. Without doubt, my own experience has made me more observant of how others respond when there is no cure. I have seen the heroic and the hopeless, the resilient and the restless, as well as the defiant and the despairing. As a pharmacist-scientist, I have also watched with dismay many patients taken advantage of by charlatans making a buck off the vulnerable among us who are on a desperate quest for relief.

As I have accumulated a progressive list of incurable diseases, I have visited an impressive array of medical specialists who investigated and prescribed interventions for each ailment. All were well-qualified professionals devoted to their calling. Still, they never spoke about the myriad ways each ailment would change my life. None inquired about or gave advice on how my ailment would affect those I lived with. Perhaps it was not their role to do so. These were all things that took time and experience to learn. I cannot recapture the time nor relive the events I now wish I handled differently. I have written to help others on their journey so they are better prepared to deal with difficult issues not often discussed—or at times poorly addressed.

I hope this work will help fellow sufferers and those who care about and for them (professionally and personally) deal with issues most health professionals don't address. Years of experience taught me things that would have been helpful early in my journey. I have written this book to help those facing a life of chronic suffering think through key issues they will need to consider—regardless of their specific ailment. I open each chapter with a vignette of my personal journey, including elements of my medical experience known to very few in my life. Personal stories are used to introduce topics because of the power of story to communicate to both the heart and the head. These experiences have also provided a strong motivation for this book. I am convinced that thriving in the face of the suffering produced by an incurable or unexplainable chronic ailment is foremost a matter of the heart. I invite you to travel through these pages with me to see if you conclude likewise.

provided a workout for my tear ducts. I began to better understand the agony of Job when he declared, "I am allotted months of emptiness, and nights of misery are apportioned to me."

Despite the physical and emotional agony, the day offered a glimmer of hope. A midmorning appointment with a renowned spinal specialist provided an opportunity to find a route to escape this persistent pain clinging to my life like barnacles on the bottom of a boat. As the hours leading up to the appointment ticked by, my hope heightened. Perhaps this journey with pain was near its conclusion. Surely, today I would get the help I needed.

"I am headed out to see a specialist. I hope he'll have ideas for getting relief from this back pain," I told my colleagues when departing my office. At the appointed hour, I entered the spinal clinic, grateful this specialist was only a short drive away. The receptionist scrunched her face when I declined to take a seat to wait. My time seemed less treasured than the specialist's, for I was the only one ready at the designated hour. After sufficient time for an unwanted level of anxiousness and annoyance to emerge, I followed a nurse down the hall to a sterile examination room. She confirmed my vital signs were stable enough to survive further waiting. The mild scent of some unknown disinfectant was all that remained as she left me in a silent chamber— providing time for me to meditate on the sad state my life had become since incessant pain parked in my back six months earlier. As I awaited the spinal specialist's assessment of the latest round of tests, and an answer as to why nothing relieved the pain, I longed for a path to escape the neurological intruder who upended my daily activities.

No aura accompanied the specialist's entrance into the exam room—just a file containing a portion of my medical records, a report from physical therapy, and images from an MRI. After bringing him up to date on how I was doing, he gave his expert opinion. Shredding hope to pieces, his words pierced like a knife into the deepest core of my being: "There is really nothing more we can do for you. You will just have to learn to live with it." Feeling as though he had punched me in the gut, I became overwhelmed with the urge to leave. Whatever else he said went unheard. I ignored the expected stop at the receptionist's desk on the way out. An unnatural darkness surrounded me as I walked from the clinic to my car. Tears clouded my vision as I drove back to my office after this appointment. This time, however, the tears were more from emotional than physical pain.

"Live with it." What would this mean for my life? I sat only when it was an absolute necessity. Other than driving, sitting was a foreign posture. It hurt too much. Typing on a keyboard balanced on top of the computer monitor—which enabled me to work standing—became a new skill. While everyone else sat, constant pain required me to remain standing at meetings. I crawled up a set of stairs on my hands and knees to our bedroom each day upon arriving home after work so I could lie down. Our children took turns eating dinner at my bedside so they wouldn't forget their father's face. My contribution to the myriad chores around our home became marginal. We canceled a planned vacation to avoid the car ride. The out-of-town funeral of a beloved family member passed unattended. Professional opportunities went by the wayside to avoid travel. What would life be like if I "lived with it"? Would it really be life?

Many Live with the Suffering of Chronic Illness with No Cure

Millions across our globe suffer with incurable ailments. Symptoms whose cause is often unknown, and whose treatment eludes the best medical minds, alter their daily lives drastically. Many are silent sufferers, their persistent agony far from obvious to those with whom they work and live life. Some live with a ticking time bomb within—dreading the next body function to go awry. Each patient has a unique experience, but all share feelings of frustration and weariness from unwelcome pathological companions who have joined them in their life journey.

The increasing life span among the general population, and our ability to aid those with declining body functions, means more people than ever are living with chronic ailments of unknown origin and/or for which there is no cure. The numbers are staggering. In the United States, two hundred new cases of multiple sclerosis are diagnosed *each week*, with almost one million people afflicted overall. Fibromyalgia, a disease leaving patients with chronic pain and fatigue, afflicts an estimated ten million people in the US, while sixty thousand people receive a diagnosis of Parkinson's disease each year. Various forms of inflammatory bowel disease affect over one and a half million Americans. Some patients manifest an incurable ailment at a young age and face a lifetime of debilitating and/or deteriorating symptoms (for example, juvenile arthritis afflicts approximately three hundred thousand in the US). Added to this are millions living with chronic pain from injuries or unknown causes. Some estimate 10 percent of the population suffers from a medical condition resulting in a disability invisible even to those who live with them. The goal of finding preventive measures and treatments will continue to be the focused effort of some of the brightest biomedical minds. Still, what are sufferers to do while they await a helpful discovery? How does one live with an ailment when there is no cure? Not just live, but also *thrive* while living with chronic illness? How do those who care about them best help?

Some incurable diseases do not produce chronic suffering. High blood pressure most often arises from unknown causes and cannot be cured. Medications for this disease reduce the risk of adverse consequences. Nevertheless, most patients with high blood pressure do not see themselves as chronic sufferers. In contrast, diseases like multiple sclerosis are incurable and marginally controlled with medications. Most patients with this disease suffer a lifetime of pain and other symptoms, including interference with important life activities. The experience of these two patient populations is quite different. Patients would not declare their high blood pressure to be life altering. Most patients with multiple sclerosis would. They and many others must live with the chronic suffering illness brings.

It is also true some diseases that cause few or no symptoms in the early years after diagnosis (such as high blood pressure and diabetes) can result in long-term organ injury, altering a patient's life dramatically. Even in their silent phase (where no symptoms are evident), patients may live with the emotional stress of knowing there is a disease lurking within their body with the potential to alter their life. For some, this knowledge itself causes unbearable distress.

Some incurable diseases are life threatening in the near term. Many forms of cancer present with minimal odds of defeating the unchecked growth of cancer cells, with survival often measured in months. The challenge this diagnosis presents is profound but quite different from those of patients facing an ailment whose slow destruction of body functions leaves sufferers with decades of debilitating symptoms. Nevertheless, many battling cancer also have life-altering experiences like those suffering from chronic ailments. Just as important is the reality that the most promising medical advances on the horizon will convert cancer to a chronic but controllable disease rather than bring a cure. Consequently, the chronicity of suffering in cancer patients is likely to be more common.

Health Professionals Are Poorly Prepared to Deal with Suffering

The expanding number of patients who are chronic sufferers has profound implications for health professionals. Health professionals are not well prepared to deal with patient suffering. Yet that is what affects patients most—not the laboratory abnormalities clinicians often try so hard to correct. The failure to train health professionals in this area of human experience means your doctor is not well prepared to help patients diagnosed with an incurable ailment deal with the profound impact of chronic suffering.

I learned to better empathize with patients in a high blood pressure clinic where I trained as a clinical pharmacist by entering into their experience. After I stressed the need for them to adhere to a low-salt diet, patients sometimes asked, "Do you know how hard that is, Doc?" Well, no, I did not. So, I went on a low-salt diet to learn what it was like. It wasn't easy. But it enabled me to engage patients with greater understanding of their plight and help them address challenges they faced to accomplish this goal since I learned to overcome some of these challenges through personal experience.

In contrast, I had no way to enter into the experience of the chronic suffering vocalized by diabetic patients with nerve pain. The first patient I cared for with this condition provided an intractable therapeutic dilemma. None of the drugs we tried relieved his pain. He told me I could not imagine what it was like to experience such a sensation in your foot all the time. He was right.

I did not know what it was like to feel a tingling pain in one of your extremities 24/7/365. Decades later, my own neuropathological companion joined me on life's journey—teaching me what it was like to experience such incessant nerve pain in an extremity. It feels like someone has inserted myriad little pins, points up, into the sole of my shoe. The worst part is that I can't make it go away. So, how do I live with it? How do I prevent it from becoming the driver of my life course? More importantly—can I thrive in the face of an added source of unremitting pain?

Every person with an incurable ailment experiences life in his or her own unique way. It would be foolhardy for anyone to write a book declaring this is what *you* should do in *your* unique circumstances. Nevertheless, I am confident there are common threads in the experience of chronic sufferers that enable me to help patients see issues they must navigate in order to thrive in the face of an incurable ailment. *How* one navigates these issues will need to be specific to their particular ailment, circumstances, and values. Nevertheless, as patients, face them we must.

The Key Challenge for Those Living with Chronic Suffering

The overarching question those of us living with chronic illnesses must face is this: How do we live with the chronic suffering of an incurable ailment without becoming obsessed with it or possessed by it?

To express it as a beneficial goal, how can we thrive despite the suffering chronic illness brings? I believe answering this question will enable us to live well. To do so means we must be intentional in our response to chronic suffering. We cannot just allow life to happen. We must think through our experience and responses to those experiences with care.

Those of us who live with an incurable ailment that alters our life course must recognize the ditches on the sides of our journey's path. Many have fallen into the ditch of obsession—becoming consumed with their ailment. For these individuals, their entire life centers on finding a solution to their suffering. In their obsessive pursuit to learn everything about their ailment and solutions for it, they often drive those most important to them to the periphery of their lives. Many seem unable to think about anything but their ailment. Their affliction defines them. They assess every minute element of their experience in terms of its potential effect on their health. The desire to avoid anything causing the slightest increase in their discomfort is the driver on their life journey. These individuals lose their joy in the simplest of activities. They view everything through the lens of their ailment and demand those around them do the same.

Others have fallen into the ditch of surrender—yielding their lives to suffering. They become hermits and withdraw from experiences that make life fulfilling and bring joy. They morph into fatalists who no longer wish to press themselves to overcome the barriers their physical ailment has produced. For them, hope has disappeared over the horizon. They define their lives by the darkness that has descended on their life through suffering.

Both ditches are easy to fall into, but neither will serve us well on the journey we call life. Neither positions us to thrive in the presence of chronic suffering. Life is more than good health. The foolish—but oft repeated—mantra, "If you don't have your health, you don't have anything," represents a depressing and narrow view of life. It also casts tens, if not hundreds, of millions who lack good health onto a path of despair. It is disheartening to encounter those with incurable ailments who have surrendered to a life of despair. The truth is, many who suffer from chronic illness have found their life journey to be fulfilling and marked by abundant joy. I am convinced this path is open to all who live with an incurable ailment that leads to chronic suffering. Yes, life is different from before chronic illness. Nevertheless, different can be fulfilling.

Managing a chronic ailment can be time consuming. Keeping track of multiple medications, making and attending various appointments with specialists, fitting innumerable lab tests into our busy schedules, and seeking as much information as possible about our disease and treatment options easily makes our head spin. It can all be quite exhausting. So much so that we can forget to manage the most important component of our lives: our hearts. Avoiding the ditches of obsessing over our illness or surrendering to suffering requires intentional management of our hearts. This is what will determine whether we thrive in the face of chronic illness.

CHAPTER 2

How to Make Your Doctor Listen: What to Say and When to Say It

My twenty-seventh year of life brought both the greatest earthly blessing and my first unwelcome permanent pathological guest. It was the year I married the woman who has proven herself a wife exceeding my dreams. Sadly, into our marital bliss came episodes of intense intestinal cramping—dropping me to my knees and writhing on the floor in pain, followed by prolonged periods in the bathroom best not described further. I concluded the first episode was food poisoning. Time showed my diagnostic skill to be lacking.

Another episode a few days after the first raised serious questions about the food poisoning hypothesis. Before long, weekly episodes became the norm—soon dotting my life several times a week. It became clear certain foods precipitated attacks, and the list of those launching an assault on my innards continued to grow. My dear wife felt petrified with each episode, thinking she had fed me something that caused my physical distress.

I began fasting on days I needed to stand before a classroom of students. The thought of making an emergency exit in the middle of a lecture was horrifying. Occasions of lengthy car rides and airplane flights joined the list of food-free days. The unexpected nature of the attacks left me imitating a seismic geologist— ever alert to activity in my gut signaling a quake was on its way. The frequency of attacks and extended periods of fasting left me physically drained. Something was seriously amiss with my gut.

My internist, a gentle Kenyan whose compassionate care remains unequaled by subsequent physicians, listened to my history with an expression of growing concern on his face. He insisted something more than food intolerance was going on. Convinced of the need to probe this further, he referred me to a gastroenterologist.

The descent of dusk matched my emotions as I arrived weeks later at the medical center for my appointment. One attack after another punctuated the preceding weeks. My gut felt like an overused punching bag. I shuddered at the thought of someone pressing on my abdomen as I slogged my way to the gastroenterology office suite. The relative quiet suggested I was one of the last patients of the day.

As I awaited my turn to get an expert opinion, the pathological possibilities rolled around inside my head. I was more anxious than hopeful. After the esteemed gastroenterologist listened to my history of symptoms, he responded by saying, "Well, everybody gets a little diarrhea every now and then." I kid you not. Those were his exact words. My first thought was that I would not classify knee-buckling abdominal pain as "a little," nor up to four debilitating attacks a week as "every now and then." My second thought was that I was wasting my time with this guy who was not taking me seriously.

Why It Seems Hard to Get Physicians to Listen

Many who journey through life with undefined or incurable ailments report the challenge of getting physicians to take their symptoms seriously. This is a long-standing problem, painfully voiced by an old Welsh proverb: "Heaven defend me from a busy doctor." The experience of visiting several clinicians before finding one who would devote the time and energy to understand a patient's troubles is all too common. It represents a source of indescribable frustration for many. Though we are inclined to ascribe these difficulties to uncaring professionals, the cause is more complex.

While working on my doctorate in clinical pharmacy, I enrolled in a course on differential diagnosis and physical assessment in the school of medicine. The most engaging faculty member in the course was a gastroenterologist. Her passion for her field and compassion for the patients she cared for was evident to all within moments of her opening words. She told us patients reporting chronic, periodic episodes of diarrhea with no clear pattern of precipitating event were among the most challenging seen by physicians. Differentiating those whose symptoms originated from gastrointestinal pathology versus those manifesting a symptom associated with a disorder outside the gut was often a frustrating experience. These symptoms are among the common reasons patients are referred to gastroenterologists—but they require significant time and skill to address. Regrettably, time is a precious commodity in most medical practices.

Physicians today often work under unreasonable time constraints and daunting patient loads. Their professional survival and personal sanity requires they cut to the chase as soon as possible in each patient encounter. Though I've been blessed with several internists over the years who somehow manage to leave me with the impression they have whatever time I need, I know the clock ticks in their head. Complex and ill-defined cases do not fit into their highly structured routine. A physician's failure to question with adequate care or dissect the clinical conundrum before them is understandable. As much as any cause, a health-system failure is what leaves many patients thinking their physician is unwilling to give them the time needed to solve their pathological puzzle.

The Disease Theory Does Not Always Serve Patients Well

A further complicating factor is that most physicians embrace the disease theory of medicine. This theoretical framework focuses effort on identifying what disease is causing a patient's symptoms—whose identity then dictates treatment. Unfortunately, the disease theory does not equip physicians to manage ailments when no definable disease is present. When a patient's chief complaint is back pain, clinicians employ tools like X-ray or MRI to look for structural injury. When such testing identifies no structural abnormality, the patient may be told everything is normal and nothing is wrong. In the clinician's mind, there is no evidence of disease. In the patient's mind, however, their pain makes it clear something is wrong and altering their life substantially. While the disease model serves medicine well in many—if not most—cases of illness, it fails to provide a roadmap for managing patients whose ailment does not meet the diagnostic criteria for a disease. It further fails to address the full spectrum of human suffering associated with physical symptoms.

The notion one cannot treat a patient without identifying the true cause of their symptoms drives the imperative to label a constellation of symptoms as a specific disease. In truth, however, diagnostic labels often do not provide a cause nor a clear connection between underlying pathology and patient symptoms. They merely allow us to put a label on the spectrum of symptoms the patient experiences. For example, the true cause of depression remains unknown. While changes in chemical messengers in the brain may occur in patients with severe depression, whether these changes represent a cause or effect of depression is open to debate. The true cause of depression remains a mystery. Despite the unknown cause, an array of drug and behavioral treatments are available to treat this mental health disorder. Likewise, the underlying cause of hypertension is unknown in most patients, leading to the classification of *essential* hypertension. Nevertheless, a variety of drugs reduce blood pressure and prevent the complications of hypertension (for example, stroke and kidney failure). Migraines represent another example of an ailment whose underlying pathology remains elusive. The many drugs with different actions on the brain that treat and prevent these crippling headaches reflects, in part, our uncertainty of their cause.

What About Symptoms of Unknown Origin?

It is also true some patients suffer symptoms not caused by a structural or functional abnormality in the body. The symptoms are no less real, but they do not arise from pathology in the organ appearing to be associated with the patient's symptoms. For example, many people experience a churning gut in response to stressful situations, such as public speaking. Some respond to their everyday environment with distressing gastrointestinal symptoms, a cycle that becomes a routine part of their lives. Others experience a rapid heart rate or debilitating headaches in response to stress. The symptoms are real and distressing to the patient, and they impair their ability to work or otherwise enjoy life. In these cases, addressing the root cause, and thereby treating the ailment, may be beyond the scope of most physicians' skills and focus. Since no clear roadmap exists for treatment when no definable disease is present, clinicians often judge such patients to have symptoms that are psychosomatic in origin and outside their ability to resolve.

Terminology for classifying patients with symptoms meeting no diagnostic criteria varies across the medical literature. Medically unexplained symptoms (MUS) is one of the most helpful and nonpejorative terms to categorize such complaints. The frequency of patients with MUS is quite high in primary care practices. For example, researchers reporting in the *International Journal of Epidemiology* estimated more than 25 percent of all primary care patients in England have unexplained symptoms of chronic fatigue, bowel distress, or pain. Many patients with MUS suffer from anxiety and/or depression and demonstrate significant improvement when treated with anxiolytics or antidepressants. Others respond to cognitive behavioral therapy. Extensive and/ or invasive testing of such patients brings inherent risks and increases healthcare costs. For this reason, psychiatric, psychological, or spiritual assessment and/or treatment for patients with MUS represents a logical next step.

Patients with MUS are best served when they are willing to consider the possibility that their symptoms are not caused by underlying organ pathology. Most of us have an aversion to considering that physical symptoms result from our response to our environment—be it job stress, deteriorating personal relationships, or a troubled past. To acknowledge such suggests we are to blame for the problem and our ailment is all in our head. Despite this concern, if we desire relief from distressing symptoms, we must be open to considering the potential of a psychogenic origin when an obvious organic explanation is absent.

It merits repeating: psychogenic does not mean the symptoms are imaginary. I once got very ill after eating scallops at a restaurant. For several decades afterward, the simple smell of scallops made me nauseated. My symptoms were quite real and reproducible. But the scallops served to another guest at my table on those occasions did not make physical contact with my body and did not directly provoke physiological changes in my gastrointestinal tract (as they had in the instance years earlier). Likewise, the rapid heart rate many people experience before public speaking is real. But nothing is awry in their heart. Treatment, therefore, must focus on a cause outside the heart.

Physicians also encounter patients who obsess over their health. These patients repeatedly present with symptoms they are certain portend the emergence of a serious illness. Such patients see the normal aches and changes in physiological functions experienced by healthy individuals as signs a catastrophic health event is just around the corner. Dealing with patients like this is frustrating and time consuming for clinicians and their staff. No amount of reassurance will allay the consuming fears of such patients. Often labeled as hypochondriacs—but more formerly categorized as illness anxiety disorder or somatic symptom disorder—these patients require intensive counseling, which is outside the scope of a normal medical practice. It is understandable when clinicians suspect individuals with MUS suffer from this ailment, and the assistance they can provide will not help.

The Danger of Rushing into Medical Labels

A further complicating factor is the substantial and inadvisable pressure for diagnostic clarity during a first patient visit. Diagnostic codes drive the American healthcare payment system, unlike some other countries in which no diagnosis on initial evaluation is more acceptable. Patients who have been struggling with symptoms are also often impatient and find imprecision in the initial assessment unacceptable. Nevertheless, clarity in diagnosis requires both time to contemplate the clinical conundrum and observation of the patient's symptoms over time. For example, a recent study published in the medical journal *Lancet Neurology* suggests some neurodegenerative diseases, such as multiple sclerosis, may provoke an emerging array of symptoms for two to five years before patients meet the disease's diagnostic criteria. This illustrates why watchful waiting often provides the wisest strategy. The calendar is one of the most important determinants for diagnostic certainty. Given time, some symptoms resolve spontaneously. In other cases, additional signs and symptoms arising over time provide diagnostic clarity.

The rush to label a patient's ailment can lead to inappropriate interventions and unnecessary stigmatization associated with certain diagnoses. Despite regulations that allow incorrect diagnoses to be corrected, removing an errant diagnosis from a patient's health record remains a challenge. This is problematic since certain diagnoses may prevent one from obtaining life insurance—or even adopting a child. Diagnostic certainty is more important than speed in pinning the cause for an ailment. An errant label for one's symptoms can be worse than no label at all.

How Do We Get Doctors to Listen?

Where do we turn when left with the sense a clinician is not taking us seriously? What tree do we shake to get the fruit of medical experience focused on the ailment that distresses our life? In essence, how do we ensure our brief encounter in a medical appointment focuses on what is important?

While open to debate, I think of myself as an intelligent person. Yet I cannot tell you how many times after visiting my internist or a specialist that my compassionate wife would ask, "Did you tell him about…?" Far too often, I would sheepishly admit I had forgotten or not gotten around to doing so in our brief encounter. She had a stroke of genius before one such visit: "Why don't you write the questions you want to ask or the things you want her to know?" Of course! Such a strategy is common sense, and it was foolish that I had not better prepared for my visits.

Do you make lists before going to the grocery store? When buying a house, did you make a list of the essential features and those preferred but not dealbreakers? Do you approach your visit with your clinician with the same careful forethought? Do you think through what you want to bring to his or her attention? Have you identified the biggest thing you want addressed (for example, my leg pain causes me to lie awake for hours most nights, desperately trying to fall asleep)? The Agency for Healthcare Research and Quality provides additional helpful tips on their website to assist patients seeking to optimize their medical visits through thoughtful preparation (see www.ahrq.gov/patients-consumers/patient-involvement/ask-your-doctor/index.html).

It is also important to consider what information you can provide your clinician in advance. If you have medical records from visits to other clinicians (including lab test results, radiological tests, etc.), sending or dropping those off in advance will optimize your visit. Handing such results to your physician at the time of your visit puts them in the difficult position of trying to absorb the mountain of documentation you've handed them at the same time they are trying to understand your verbalized history.

Recognizing the limited time a clinician spends with each patient, we must seize the initiative, think in advance about what to communicate, and make sure we do so. Why waste time hearing my potassium level is normal if I don't have time to get to the fact that the bottom of my right foot feels like I have a bad sunburn—even though the shower is the only place I've been barefoot for six months?

There are key things any clinician needs to assess about reported symptoms: onset, frequency, severity, and precipitating and/or alleviating factors. When did the symptoms begin (onset)? How often do they occur (frequency)? While clinicians are prone to measuring severity on an arbitrary scale of one to ten, it is far better to express symptoms in terms of how they impair our ability to complete normal daily activities. It also is important to know what activities worsen symptoms, in addition to anything we have found that provides relief.

Placing the symptoms in the context of our life activity is essential to communicating its importance. By context, I mean the impact symptoms have on our life. But we often stop at mentioning symptoms and do not tell about the impact they have on our daily lives. Talking with our clinicians about this and other elements of our symptoms will allow them to understand the significance of the ailment on our life. But we shouldn't waste our time or theirs by guessing. Keeping a diary of symptoms and associated activities for a meaningful period will provide important data (and there are technological tools to help you do this, such as health apps for smartphones). We can then use this data to create a concise summary to show the care we have taken to assess our symptoms.

For example, "These headaches began about six months ago. I have kept a diary for sixty days and had a severe headache at least twice a week for the past two months, usually lasting about three hours. I am unable to read, work on a computer, or do much of anything. When they occur during the workday—which all but a few have—I have to go home and lie down. Over-the-counter medications don't seem to shorten the duration or reduce the severity of the pain." Now we've done an important part of the work for our healthcare provider—which saves valuable time—and laid out the impact on our life.

What to Do When They Still Won't Listen

An ailment impairing the ability to work or enjoy normal daily activities should be seen as needing attention by even the busiest of clinicians. When we have communicated carefully and our clinician seems to ignore our stated concern, we need to redirect the encounter back to the main issue: "Perhaps I have not communicated very well, but this is the most significant thing relating to my health right now. I need help getting this problem under control." If such redirection doesn't work, do not hesitate to be frank: "It doesn't seem like you think this merits attention. Could you tell me why?" The response we receive may be comforting or signal the need to look for a new healthcare provider.

Firing your physician, or other healthcare provider, is more than distasteful—it seems like a divorce. Nevertheless, a clinician must engender trust and confidence from their patients to fulfill their clinical responsibility. If trust and confidence evaporates or is never gained, they cannot fulfill their role. Many people can give advice on when to find another physician. An internet search for "fire your doctor" will reveal more hits than you could read. This obviously is not a rare dilemma.

As with other relationships in life, severing a relationship with a healthcare provider should be an uncommon response. Better to improve the interactions we are having than starting over with a new provider. Most people enter the practice of medicine with a strong desire to help people. Over time, however, financial and bureaucratic hurdles may dull this honorable motivation. Like most with careers devoted to serving others, clinicians sometimes need reminders of their high calling. They will most often rise to the better nature of their profession when challenged. If not, it may be time to sever the relationship.

Searching for a new healthcare provider can be frustrating. If you do change your primary care provider, identify the characteristics most important to you in a clinician. The U.S. Department of Health and Human Services provides helpful tips for selecting a physician (see healthfinder.gov/HealthTopics/Category/doctor-visits/regular-check-ups/choosing-a-doctor-quick-tips) as do some consumer groups. Review one or more of these lists before you begin your search. Then take advantage of family, social, and professional connections to get recommendations. Be sure to ask why they love their physician, as a friend's priorities for a clinician may be different from yours.

When changing specialists, your primary care provider is the best source for a recommendation. Communicate why you left dissatisfied and what you want in a new specialist. The direct referral of your primary care provider may give you quicker access for a first appointment with a specialist. If a diagnosis of your condition is known, patient support groups are also a helpful source for recommendations. The Genetic and Rare Diseases Information Center of the National Institutes of Health provides helpful resources for those searching for clinicians experienced with rare diseases (see rarediseases.info.nih.gov/guides/pages/25/how-to-find-a-disease-specialist).

Feeling that clinicians are not taking your concerns seriously is frustrating and an all too common complaint. With appropriate proactive steps, we can seize the initiative and assure we receive the best care possible.

CHAPTER 3

What to Do When Doctors Don't Know How to Help

I won't share the words of my internist when I told him the response of the gastroenterologist who declared, "Everyone gets a little diarrhea every now and then." It wasn't foul; it's just best not put to writing. However, I am confident this specialist never received further referrals from my dear physician. He set me up with another gastroenterologist, who he was certain would exhibit better clinical judgment. I hoped he was correct.

Weeks later, I sat in the waiting room for another late-afternoon appointment with a gastroenterologist. My expectations were not high. I just wanted someone who would not dismiss my complaints. Gratitude rose within me when this one listened with care to my history. He expressed serious concern about the frequency and severity of my attacks. He focused particular attention on the nutritional implications of my frequent avoidance of food. After a brief physical, he expressed his concurrence that food intolerance was not the root of the problem—rather it was an aggravating factor. He recommended further tests, including the dreaded sticking of a tube up where no man should go. Why anyone would want to do this for a living remains a mystery to me.

The late-night pretreatment bowel evacuation process before the test made me more miserable. I thought I couldn't have been more uncomfortable when I arrived for the test the next morning. But after he inserted the tube and inflated my bowel with air, I learned the meaning of true misery. The air provoked intestinal cramping of epoch proportions—so much that the gastroenterologist cut the procedure short because of the level of my discomfort. He declared he had never seen a patient cramp with such severity, though I didn't feel it an honor to be so exceptional. After I occupied the office bathroom for an inordinate period, my wife steadied me as we walked back to our vehicle. I left concerned that the shortened procedure would leave the diagnosis unresolved.

We scheduled a follow-up appointment for a few weeks later to get the results of the biopsy he snipped before withdrawing the intrusive snake from my innards. He told us his visual evaluation revealed minor inflammation of the bowel wall but no evidence of ulcerative colitis or Crohn's disease—the two most common inflammatory bowel diseases. At my return visit, he said the biopsy revealed a rare form of colitis— one associated with a thickening of collagen in the bowel wall. Mine was extensive. The good news? I had a real disease. The bad news? No one knew how to treat it.

Like any biomedical scientist worth their salt, my first response was to perform an extensive literature search. Sifting through endless pages of hefty medical journals for countless hours, I found fewer than forty cases of this disease reported to date. There was not a single study to determine the effectiveness of any form of treatment. None. There were a few case reports describing efforts to use drugs that had helped treat other inflammatory bowel diseases. These reports were not encouraging. I felt like a man trapped in a familiar room with no escape route.

Facing the Trauma of a Rare Disease Diagnosis

Many ailments exist that affect small numbers of patients, but we know little to nothing about effective treatment for them. If all the people in the US with a rare disorder joined hands, they would circle our globe one and a half times. It is distressing to receive a diagnosis only to learn no known treatment exists. Patients express an overwhelming sense of powerlessness to combat an enemy who has raised its ugly head within their bodies. Should we succumb to its many manifestations or identify beachheads on which to stand to stave off this invader?

There are key steps toward a path of living well in this situation. It begins by dealing with the emotional trauma such news brings. Before the condition is defined, an inner sense exists that "this too shall pass." Once defined with the label of a disease, however, we come to grips with the realization an unexpected turn has occurred on our life's journey, causing our plans for the future to crumble. No obvious escape route from this unwanted path makes the impact more profound.

Receiving the diagnosis of an incurable ailment may feel like watching a bridge on the road before us collapse into the valley below. Our first response is shock. Then comes disorientation, as the path we thought we'd travel is no longer available, leaving us uncertain where to turn. Once the reality sinks in, we realize we need to chart a new course, one quite different from what we expected. It will change what we thought the future would be. How do we respond to such news in a way that allows us to move forward in our lives? How do we chart a new course?

When possible, avoid life-altering decisions when pierced through by emotional trauma—be it trauma of the death of a life companion or an ominous diagnosis. I have known of individuals who immediately ended relationships so as not to burden the other person with their newly diagnosed disease. Others made a job change to accommodate what they expected to be their future level of incapacitation. Give the truth time to sink in, seek wise counsel if needed, but don't jump ship at the first sound that trouble may be around the bend. Many have charted a path of living well in the face of chronic illness, and we can learn from their examples.

Then, once the news has sunk in—giving you time to take stock of this new reality—education should be the next order of business. Sometimes being a passive patient makes sense, such as when illness impairs cognitive ability and one cannot think straight, but this is not one of those times. Just as a collapsed bridge would draw us to a map to examine alternative routes from the one we were traveling, we need information to help us chart a new course in life to account for the altered future we are facing. The education must focus on both developing a greater self-awareness and understanding the ailment itself.

Become a Student of Yourself

First, we need to get a clear picture of how this pathological companion who has joined us in the saddle is changing our ride through life. As no two people are alike, the manifestations of ailments vary from patient to patient. We need to become students of our body. This ailment is now a part of us. We need to work at identifying precipitating factors, actions that bring relief, and the normal oscillating pattern of the ailment. Keeping a health diary for a period to become familiar with how this ailment affects our body will be very important. We may benefit from someone else who can help us observe the personality of this disorder afflicting us. My wife did not have the benefit of the formal training in patient assessment and differential diagnosis I received. Nevertheless, she is a superb observer of her husband and has often been quicker to notice patterns and precipitating factors of my ailments.

In *Poor Richard's Almanack*, Benjamin Franklin declared, "There are three things extremely hard, steel, a diamond, and to know one's self." While likely referring to inner character and its manifestations, Franklin's dictum also rings true in understanding our physical selves. It takes work to develop a full portrait of how an ailment changes the contours of our lives. Those contours will be both physical and psychological as well as relational.

I took years to realize how my intestinal ailment influenced our family when we traveled. Since I could experience a colitis attack with little to no warning, I became tense if we were far from a bathroom. That was frequently the case when visiting family, which often involved driving hundreds of miles through Canadian farmland where rest stops were rare (trees were also infrequent). A colitis attack on the road would have been more than inconvenient. Since food often precipitated an attack, I fasted while traveling, which left me weak. Sadly, my family often bore the brunt of my tension. Suffice it to say, I was a less than desirable traveling companion. I focused on the physical impact of my ailment and just getting through each day, whether traveling or not. Consequently, I did not take the needed care to assess the emotional impact on those I loved and on me. Time—and a patient wife— eventually corrected this deficiency on my part. But I live with the regret of years of self-centered ignorance.

Those of us who experience incurable ailments owe it to those we love, and even those with whom we casually interact, to learn how this intruder affects how we engage others—and its impact on their lives. Studies have found the quality of life for spouses and partners is sometimes poorer than the quality of life for the patient with chronic illness. This reflects the profound effect of our illness on others. Loved ones not only experience disruption of their lives but may also respond with anxiety and depression. Family and friends want to ease our burden, so we should not increase theirs through our poor emotional responses. This requires careful reflection and open communication to understand the interplay between our ailment and our interaction with others. Living well hinges on maintaining healthy relationships with those who are important to us. Frequent slices of humble pie are often necessary to achieve this goal.

Learn About the Disease

The second educational focus is about the disease—how it manifests itself in most people, what normal progression looks like, and what options exist for treatment. Learning as much as we can about the ailment is important—including how clearly we fit or do not fit the diagnostic criteria. Shouldn't we leave this to our physician? We could, but there are many reasons we should not. If there are no effective treatments for our illness, it is likely the disorder is infrequent among the population. This means our physician has seen few, if any, cases. Consequently, they are likely limited in their knowledge of the ailment. If they are a specialist, their knowledge base will be more expansive—perhaps to the point that they are an expert in the particular ailment. Even in these cases, it behooves us to learn as much as practical about the ailment, for two reasons:

Misdiagnoses occur. It is an unfortunate reality. Many factors contribute to its occurrence, but one need not search long or far to find patients whose self-education led them to suspect an errant diagnosis, one subsequently confirmed as erroneous by other specialists. A recent survey conducted by Multiplesclerosis.net found 42 percent of patients with multiple sclerosis initially received a misdiagnosis—erroneously labeling them with another condition. This illustrates the high frequency of misdiagnosis in patients with uncommon ailments. Many people give the testimony of finding a path to better living by having an errant diagnosis corrected.

Outcomes are better. Numerous studies show patients who understand their diabetes, high blood pressure, asthma, or other diseases have better health outcomes. We have every reason to believe the same to be true for other ailments. Understanding the underlying ailment enables patients to know what to expect, when to seek medical help for new symptoms, and potential means of reducing the impact of the ailment.

Self-education should not create the delusion we will become a self-made diagnostician or that we will trump experts. While taking psychology as a freshman in college, I self-diagnosed several disorders during the semester. I had none of the disorders. Yet a little knowledge can be a dangerous thing. We should keep this in mind while learning about a newly diagnosed disease or evolving constellation of symptoms. No amount of internet searching will replace the intensive didactic and experiential education—and years of working with patients—of a skilled clinician. Nevertheless, this education can arm patients with important questions to raise with their healthcare provider.

I know little about home construction or fixing problems with an existing home. Still, I am in my home every day and have observed its details more intensely than a repairman on a first visit. On occasion, a home repair specialist has proposed a fix for a problem, but their idea for a solution made little sense to me. Admitting my lack of specialist knowledge, I have had them try their proposed fix for the problem. Sometimes, my hunch proved correct, while their expert diagnosis and remedy was wrong. This experience, however, does not make me a home repair expert.

In the same respect, as patients we know our body—specifically how symptoms wax and wane. Just because we are not an expert clinician does not mean our insights lack value. By educating ourselves as much as practical, we can more effectively collaborate with our healthcare providers.

As patients, we should identify in advance what information we want to obtain as we seek to educate ourselves about our ailment. Otherwise, it is easy to drown in the sea of information available in the health arena. We need to recognize that websites often post bad health information. Consequently, it is essential to think about how to assess the trustworthiness of information surfaced from an internet search. The Access to Credible Genetics Resource Network has created a helpful tool patients can use to think through the credibility of posted health information (www. trustortrash.org/#). Some sites scrutinize posted information by vetting with recognized experts (for example, WebMD, Mayo Clinic). There are also sites that provide carefully evaluated information, but also post less reliable blogs or personal testimonies.

Questions to probe in an online search include:

What is known about the natural course of the disease or pattern of the ailment?

This will indicate what to expect as the ailment progresses. In addition, a significant deviation from the normal pattern may suggest a questionable diagnosis. It will also help patients think about life adjustments to consider as the ailment progresses. Understanding the natural course of the ailment can help identify symptoms that should prompt medical attention.

Disease-specific patient advocacy groups are often a helpful source of information regarding the normal patterns of a disease. Their websites are an accessible source of material summarizing the current state of knowledge about the disease. The best groups are those that include an expert advisory panel to assess the accuracy of information provided. You should be cautious about sites and groups that provide information but lack such an advisory panel. The National Institutes of Health websites also contain helpful information on many diseases.

Is there any evidence for effective treatment?

For many ailments, no effective treatments exist. The Committee on Drugs of the American Academy of Pediatrics found that most rare disease patients receive drugs approved by the Food and Drug Administration (FDA) for a different disorder. Knowing about these available options will help lead patients to an informed decision. Patient advocacy groups can often be a helpful source of information about treatment options. These groups can also provide information about ongoing clinical trials of potential therapies. However, health experts have expressed concern about the financial conflicts of interest among patient advocacy groups. A recent report published in the *New England Journal of Medicine* noted that many advocacy groups receive significant support (some as much as 50 percent of their revenue) from pharmaceutical companies who produce products marketed or undergoing clinical trials for the disease on which these groups focus. While a conflict of interest does not negate the value of information provided, advocacy groups should be transparent about their sources for support. Kaiser Health News has created a database, Pre$cription For

Power (https://khn.org/patient-advocacy/#), enabling interested parties to find what companies are supporting specific patient advocacy groups and at what dollar amount.

What are the most troubling symptoms, and is there a physiological basis for an unproven treatment?

People with rare disorders often face a painful reality—there are no treatments proven to be effective for their disease. This does not mean, however, that there is no hope for relief from troubling symptoms. As noted physician Sir William Osler declared, "Medicine is a science of uncertainty and an art of probability." The uncertainty of the best treatment option means the physician needs to apply the breadth of his or her knowledge to develop a rational, personalized approach for a patient. Clinicians will sometimes try medications to tackle the most troubling symptoms based on their knowledge of physiology and pharmacology.

It may make sense to try a treatment found to work on related ailments. I faced the reality of no approved treatment on the market when diagnosed with a rare form of colitis. My gastroenterologist suggested we try a course of treatments approved for other forms of inflammatory bowel disease. Such use is referred to as "off-label"—meaning the FDA approved the drug for some disease, but not the specific application for a particular patient. In my case, such medications proved ineffective in reducing the frequency or severity of attacks.

After years of ineffective treatments, I sat next to a gastroenterologist as part of a panel reviewing grants for the National Institutes of Health. He struggled with an inflammatory bowel disease for which there are several FDA-approved treatments. He also cared for several patients with the same rare form of colitis as mine. Consistent with my experience, each of these patients reported attacks provoked by an increasing number of food substances. He suspected food in the small intestine was stimulating the release of bile salts and provoking the symptoms. With this hypothesis in mind, he treated his patient cohort with an agent that binds bile salts and found it dramatically reduced the frequency and severity of their attacks. When I tried a course of the same medication, I too experienced a dramatic reduction of attacks. Stopping the drug for a period precipitously increased the number of my attacks—which then decreased when I restarted the drug.

This is an example of a clinician taking his or her knowledge of patient symptoms, precipitating factors, and physiology to deploy a drug for an unproven purpose. It shows the value of the freedom clinicians have to use drugs for ailments other than those approved by the FDA. Current laws allow licensed prescribers to prescribe a medication that is FDA approved for any legitimate medical purpose. This freedom is too often compromised by the increasing scrutiny of insurance companies, which may refuse to provide coverage for an off-label use. Importantly, a study published in the *Journal of Clinical Epidemiology* found some drugs used off-label for an ailment are actually more effective than the FDA-approved drugs for treatment of that ailment. Such off-label use was life transforming for me. I went from about four attacks per week to only four attacks of colitis in the first four months of treatment. I was able to introduce foods into my diet that I had avoided for years. Travel was no longer an anxiety-producing event.

If you decide to consider using a drug not yet studied and approved for your ailment, it is extremely important—as for all drug use—to identify criteria to determine if you are benefiting from the drug. This may be challenging for some patients. Nevertheless, it is essential to judge whether a treatment is beneficial. Consensus reports by medical professional organizations provide goals for treating a patient with high blood pressure or elevated cholesterol, but setting targets for symptoms that come and go—or vary in intensity over time—is more difficult. Despite this challenge, it is important to have an open and frank discussion with a clinician about the specific goals for any therapy. Modern pharmaceuticals save lives and make life more bearable for millions of people. At the same time, all drug therapy comes with risk (not to mention financial costs). It is unwise to remain on drug therapy without clear evidence of effectiveness.

The strongest evidence of effectiveness may be through a period of a drug holiday. Stopping treatment for a period will determine if symptoms recur and are

- interventions for which data does not exist
to assess its safety or efficacy for the ailment

FDA-approved drugs, dietary supplements, acupuncture, and all other interventions will fall into one of these three categories for a specific ailment.

Many claims exist that dietary supplements, acupuncture, and other interventions are effective for a host of ailments. In fact, no dietary supplement has gained approval to treat any disease, and the evidence for other modalities of treatment are sparse. Before trying such interventions, patients should determine what evidence exists for the value of the intervention— whether a plausible explanation exists for why it might be effective in treating a particular ailment. One can always find an explanation somewhere, but the key is whether it is plausible. Does it make sense based on our knowledge of physiology and the nature of the substance? Some explanations that rationalize a dietary supplement's ability to treat specific ailments are sheer nonsense. They reveal the author possesses no meaningful knowledge of physiology. The internet has provided a broad reach for the snake oil salesmen of our day, and patients should be wary of these kinds of online claims.

Patients who decide to try a nontraditional treatment for their ailment need to identify how to assess the impact of the treatment on their specific ailment. Otherwise, patients risk long-term treatment with an intervention that provides no benefit and therefore only puts them at risk for adverse effects. I have consulted with patients who take ten or more dietary supplements to treat a disorder without any measures identified to assess the supplement's effectiveness. Their purchases improved the profits of the manufacturers but provided no way to assess whether the patient was benefiting.

Serious and valid concerns exist about the quality of products commonly labeled as dietary or nutritional supplements. These products do not fall under the same regulatory requirements as prescription and nonprescription medications. Consequently, studies have repeatedly shown misrepresentation of the contents of such products, as well as contamination with harmful substances (for example, heavy metals like lead, mercury, and arsenic), or even prescription drugs not noted on the label. Before using products of this nature, investigate the quality of the product. The United States Pharmacopeia (USP) is a nonprofit organization that sets standards for the quality of medicinal products. Manufacturers can earn the USP Verified Dietary Supplements seal of approval by meeting their standards. Consumers can be confident in the quality of products with this distinctive mark. The USP does not assess the safety or efficacy of the product in humans, but this seal shows the manufacturer meets the USP quality standards for production (such as quality control tests to assure the accuracy of the amount listed on the label and a product that does not contain harmful contaminants).

The Need for a Team Approach

Patients with diseases lacking known effective treatments are more likely to visit multiple clinicians for help in managing their chronic illness. This has become common with the growth of alternative medicine practitioners (such as naturopathic). The scenario of multiple professionals managing the same ailment is a setup for problems and a source of significant frustration for clinicians.

In my younger years, I sought to improve my bowling skill—with a goal of achieving a specific three-game set average score. I received advice from numerous excellent bowlers, both formally and informally. One was an elderly man whose health did not allow him to bowl anymore but who was an outstanding coach. In one session, he looked at me with frustration and said, "You are getting advice from too many people, and we're working at cross purposes. You need to pick one coach and let them guide you." There was more than one way to improve my bowling skill, but as my coach wisely counseled, to travel on multiple paths at the same time was foolish.

The same is true with our health—especially when faced with an ailment lacking an obvious direction for treatment. A team approach often provides optimal care. However, a team represents a group of individuals who work *together* for the same goal, with each knowing their specific role. Disconnected individuals working in isolation to manage our health is not a team—it's an unruly mob! We need to pick a "coach" in whom we have confidence and work with them to manage our health. Above all, we must not hide from one professional our engagement with other professionals to address our health needs. The potential for interactions between medications and herbal products, for example, is too great to risk the consequences of withholding from our prescriber information about our use of such products. If we lack confidence in a clinician's ability to guide our treatment effectively, then we should search for one in whom we can place our confidence.

Receiving a diagnosis of an ailment that lacks proven treatment is an unsettling experience. Yet it is a path millions have walked. A thoughtful approach to this unexpected diversion in our expected life course is essential to thriving on our journey.

CHAPTER 4

How to Live with Pain That Won't Go Away

Who would have thought picking up a pair of socks could alter your life? Nonetheless, this simple act on a November morning turned my daily experience on its head. I arrived in the historic Georgetown district of Washington, DC, the night before to serve on a panel for the National Institutes of Health. The group would devote the next two days to reviewing grants from scientists across the country. Each grant would be given a score used in part to determine whether the proposed project received funding. Such decisions could make or break the career of the applicants. I have always had some trepidation commenting on proposals, knowing the impact my assessment could have on the applicant's future. My mind focused on this duty as I readied myself for the day.

In the dim light of dawn, I bent over to reach into my suitcase for a pair of socks. As though captured in the grip of a sumo wrestler, my lower back seized with intense pain. Straightening up demanded an incredible measure of fortitude to push through the agony. Putting on and tying my shoes left me near tears. Every step, even in slow motion, caused my face to contort into a wince. The shake of the elevator at each floor before my destination almost took my breath away. During the two days of panel discussion, the nerve signals in my back screamed in my body like a tornado siren. The journey home via taxi, airplane, and car was like traveling through a series of torture chambers.

The pain progressed down my leg and left me unable to sit without intense agony. Several days of muscle relaxants and pain relievers only induced drowsiness. A course of physical therapy likewise failed to forestall my worsening pain. Failing to improve with the usual interventions, I received a referral to a spinal center that, among other accolades, cared for the elite athletes of the Detroit Red Wings and the Detroit Lions. If they could handle the trauma incurred by professional athletes, I figured the pain that resulted from picking up a pair of socks from a suitcase should be a cinch for them to manage. This turned out to be nothing more than wishful thinking on my part.

Numerous additional interventions proved unsuccessful in halting my unremitting pain. Many of these attempts left me, at least temporarily, in worse shape. Naturally, I hesitated when I considered the next recommendation to address my pain. When the specialist rendered the unhappy verdict that neither the art nor science of medicine had anything further to offer (as you may recall from chapter 1), a life of constant pain with its associated limitations appeared to be inescapable. I joined the millions of people who live with chronic pain and understood what C. S. Lewis meant when he said, "Pain insists upon being attended to."

The Problem of Pain

Pain affects more people than cancer, diabetes, and heart disease combined. Estimates from the National Institutes of Health indicate over twenty-five million adults have experienced pain *every day* for the preceding three months. The costs of chronic pain in America in terms of healthcare and lost wages exceeds $500 billion annually. But the true human toll associated with chronic pain is immeasurable. Promising careers ended. Marriages dissolved. Families shipwrecked. Bankruptcy incurred. Lives ended by the sufferer's own hands. Add to this list a thousand lesser impacts on the daily lives of millions. The inescapable reality that pain is now a constant companion can lead to despair. Some individuals give up all hope of finding joy and fulfillment in life. They manifest what psychologists call *learned helplessness*.

Learned helplessness can occur in people who repeatedly experience pain or other noxious stimuli they cannot avoid. This leads to a sense of hopelessness— whereby the person ceases any effort to mitigate the discomfort. They surrender to sadness, experience increasing physical symptoms of illness, and give way to a pervasive negative view on life.

Facing the reality of a life of pain, my mind recounted the experience of an acquaintance named Mike. He was a strapping specimen of manhood used to physical activity, but an injury left him with excruciating back pain. When we met, he had been living with constant pain for several years. Despite evaluations by specialists near and far, our first handshake revealed him to be a man in a fragile state. Every move of his body molded his face into a grimace. Just the parting of his teeth to annunciate words appeared to intensify his pain. No one was able to offer him relief. A few years after our first meeting, Mike opted for the only source of relief he felt remained—he ended his life. With a similar road of incessant pain lying before me, how could I prevent myself from spiraling into a similar state of despair?

The words of the specialist to which I referred in chapter 1, "There is really nothing more we can do for you, you will just have to learn to live with it," were unfortunate. A helpless patient with an unhelpful physician can give rise to a sense of hopelessness. It was true he could see no path to remove my pain. Numerous tests provided no clue to a repairable cause. The various injections and other efforts had not eliminated my pain. Despite these failures, there were steps available to help me better live with pain. Occupational therapists could offer help to arrange my workspace to make standing a better way to work. A different vehicle might make transportation more comfortable. Physical therapy could strengthen core muscles so fewer activities would aggravate the persistent pain I faced. Despite the profound changes pain brought with it, there was hope interventions could improve my life experience. This was the message the specialist should have delivered.

While pain might be inescapable, the extent of its impact is far from inevitable. Life would be different without it, but that does not mean life will be unfulfilling and absent of joy. There are key steps for those living with chronic pain to ensure they experience life to the fullest, despite the persistent pulse of pain.

The Cause of Chronic Pain Is Commonly Unknown

Those who live with chronic pain of unknown cause must realize their case is common. Clinicians are unable to pinpoint a definitive cause in most patients with chronic pain. This does not mean there was not a cause, but evidence of the cause has faded over time or, if remaining, eludes our ability to probe the human body.

Most people are familiar with the prehistoric monument in Wiltshire, England, known as Stonehenge. The most casual observer of this ring of stones, each of which stands about thirteen feet tall and weighs twenty-five tons, senses their purposeful arrangement. Someone put these stones in their place. Archaeologists estimate construction occurred between 3,000 and 2,000 BC. But who erected this monument, and how they did so, remains unknown. The purpose, process, and people behind this arrangement of large stones have vanished over time.

In like manner, the cause of the physiological or anatomical alterations leading to chronic pain is no longer discernible in most patients. Something changed in their body that resulted in chronic pain. They may or may not associate its initiation with a specific event, such as a fall or other accident. But the structural injury leading to pain that persisted beyond the expected healing time went undetected and is no longer evident. Like a stone provoking concentric ripples across the surface of a pond, the root cause of the ripple of pain in their body has vanished from sight. Something caused the pain—but its provocateur has fled the scene. This is the common plight of people with chronic pain. If this describes your experience, it is not some strange abnormality. The lack of an identifiable cause does not invalidate a patient's experience of pain.

This is a critical issue for patients, as well as those most important to them, to grasp. We live in a world governed by cause and effect. This universal law states every effect has a definite cause. Whether they consciously embrace this universal law or not, people will question subjective experiences when the cause is indiscernible. Pain is subjective and not directly observable. It is a symptom reported by patients—as opposed to a sign like temperature, heart rate, or blood pressure. When the best of medical technology and skill is unable to find a cause for a patient's reported pain, others (including clinicians, family, and employers) will often question whether their account of symptoms is valid. This questioning only adds to the suffering these patients experience.

It is also true some people claim to be in pain as a manipulative effort to get things. Any emergency room physician can recount experiences of patients coming to the emergency room complaining of intense pain from minor injuries in a scheme to get potent narcotic pain relievers. I have known addicts who repeatedly faked or self-inflicted injuries to acquire opioid prescriptions. Caseworkers for social services could entertain us with stories of people reporting incapacitating pain as an effort to get unmerited disability status—and the regular disability check this status will provide. These, and other sad examples, have created a suspicious perspective in our society toward those describing chronic pain of unknown cause. Understanding the nature of chronic pain is the only way to dispel such suspicions (see the upcoming section on the nature of pain).

Accepting Pain as a Companion on Our Life Journey

Accepting enduring pain as the new normal for our life does not mean we jettison hope of relief, nor that life cannot be fulfilling. Medical advances may provide a clearer understanding of the cause of our pain or treatment options unknown today. Remaining alert to such advances makes perfect sense. But for many, there comes a time to cease the aggressive pursuit of a cure—a pursuit that can be all consuming. Instead, the focus becomes management of pain to enable the richest life possible under the circumstances. Enemies we are unable to conquer can often be held at bay. The tension of their presence will not fully abate, but their impact can be reduced, and life can be rich.

We experienced repeated drills in my elementary school where we were required to go into the hall away from windows and sit with our head between our legs. What protection this maneuver would give in the face of a nuclear bomb I never could grasp, but the acute reality of the Soviet Union's nuclear arsenal had a profound impact on our lives. People stored food and water in their basements, schools and various institutions did drills, and in many other ways the nuclear threat influenced how we lived our lives as Americans. Eventually, nuclear weapon possession by enemies became the new normal. While the devastating potential of an attack has not lessened, we have adjusted, and the threat has become less life altering for the average American. Although the threat has not disappeared, we learned how to hold it at bay, and its impact on the routine of life has diminished.

Those who face the hard reality of enduring pain can find ways to reduce its intrusion on their daily lives and make its presence tolerable. Indeed, to live well we *must* find ways to declaw this enemy groping at our nervous system. While its presence may be inescapable, pain need not rule a person's life. Will it alter our life in measurable ways? Yes. But rule our life? No! In other words, the first step may be this: jettison the notion that pain-free is the only avenue to living well. If we view complete escape from pain as the only acceptable state of being, life will indeed be intolerable for many.

Learn About the Nature of Pain

When we come to grips with the reality that our pain will not disappear, what do we do next? Chronic pain is arguably the ultimate example of a disease requiring careful self-management. This is because pain perception is inextricably linked to our emotional selves. Clinical studies have repeatedly demonstrated the profound impact of mood, conditioning, and beliefs on the experience of pain. While many bristle at suggestions that their pain is in their head, pain always involves the mind. This does not suggest the one describing pain is faking it. But the mind plays an important role in both our perception of and response to pain. Those living with chronic pain should receive the link between the mind and pain experience as empowering. Apart from medications and external interventions, we have the ability to modulate our pain experience.

For example, people living with chronic pain will often experience increased pain during times of stress. Learning how to reduce stress, or to better cope with its presence in our lives, can reduce pain. Similarly, anxiety can provoke pain in patients with ailments like trigeminal neuralgia (painful attacks arising from a misfiring of the trigeminal nerve in the jaw). Addressing the underlying causes of anxiety can reduce the episodes of painful attacks in such patients. In essence, we must learn to deal with our pain holistically to hold this enemy at bay. Understanding pain and its causes will empower us to do so, developing an individualistic approach to manage the pain in our lives.

Chronic pain is also very different from acute pain. Acute pain presents important warning signals telling us something needs attention right away (get your hand out of that flame!). Chronic pain appears to involve pain signals that don't turn off when they should, as well as changes in the signals dampening pain. Patient experiences of and responses to chronic pain also differ from those of acute pain. Most people have only experienced acute pain. When they equate our chronic pain to their experience with acute pain, the result will be—at the least—misconceptions about our experience. Developing the ability to explain the differences between these two types of pain will enable us to educate others in our life (see notes for a link to a helpful video on this topic).

Seek Help from Those Who Specialize in Pain Management

Most primary care providers are adept at treating acute pain. Management of chronic pain is more difficult, requiring the expertise of those specializing in pain management. A multidisciplinary approach—meaning involvement of individuals from a variety of health professions—is often necessary for optimal treatment of patients with chronic pain. It is difficult to overstate the importance and value of receiving care from pain management specialists.

The renowned physician Sir William Osler said, "The practice of medicine is an art based on science." Experience is an essential supplement to knowledge in the art of medicine. Those specializing in pain medicine have focused their energy and training toward honing those skills essential for effective management of chronic pain. They have experience managing such patients far surpassing the experience of primary care providers. Their professional toolkit will hold a more diverse array of options for helping us manage our pain.

Unfortunately, pain specialists are not readily accessible for many people. For example, the physician registry for the American Academy of Pain Medicine lists only five cities in the entire state of Indiana, where I live, with a pain specialist in practice. It is understandable when patients abandon the idea of seeing such specialists if they are too far away. Nevertheless, if the foreseeable future involves living with chronic pain, the investment to travel and be evaluated by a qualified specialist is likely to provide greater benefit to us than any vacation for which we might spend similar resources. Advances in telehealth are likely to enhance accessibility of such specialists soon. In the meantime, a local primary care provider may be willing to provide regular management through cooperation with a distant specialist. Many primary care providers make such arrangements for patients with rare diseases.

Establish Realistic Goals for Pain Relief

As indicated earlier, there comes a point in time to recognize that eradicating pain is an unrealistic near-term goal. This does not require surrendering to the suffering chronic pain produces. It does mean establishing new goals to enable us to live life to the fullest extent possible. This should begin with identifying the most important areas where pain interferes with meaningful activities in our life, then learning about options for reducing pain during these activities. We also need to think about what price we are willing to pay to get pain relief. Many have found a measure of pain is better than the side effects associated with maximal relief from potent pain relievers. Is achieving a pain-free experience worth the price if relieving pain comes with diminishing cognitive ability to the degree we cannot enjoy the things in life we value?

We are all familiar with the common question of rating our pain on a scale of one to ten. While such approaches increase the attention healthcare providers give to patient pain, managing chronic pain by such an arbitrary—and nonreproducible—scale is not in the best interests of patients. Fortunately, chronic pain management is evolving to focus more on functional goals rather than numerical pain rankings.

For example, I identified being able to drive without excruciating pain as a key goal—yet I was unwilling to accept drowsiness or dulled cognitive ability to obtain this goal through medication. Ultimately, I purchased an SUV of substantial height that did not require lowering myself into the seat of a car. While this did not eliminate pain upon sitting, it reduced the intensity so the act of driving no longer induced tears. It required a financial investment, but in the long term, this was among the best investments I made in life. In fact, refraining from sitting in a car (as opposed to an SUV or minivan) did more to improve my pain than any form of physical therapy or medication.

The ability to stand comfortably while working was another high-priority goal I identified when it became clear chronic pain would be a part of my daily experience. Investing in a standing desk for my computer, and a thick pad on which to stand to cushion my feet, made my workday much more bearable. Consulting with an occupational therapist can help create a work environment that optimizes functionality and reduces pain. Many large employers have a unit devoted to providing ergonomically improved work environments for employees—especially those with disabilities.

Pain screams loudest when all else has gone quiet. This means sleep is often elusive for those living with chronic pain. Sleeping through the night has been such a rarity for me that I announce its occurrence to my wife with greater surprise than finding a four-leaf clover. Adequate sleep is very important to our overall health, and addressing pain's negative effect on sleep should be a goal for anyone living with chronic pain.

A pain specialist can work with patients to establish achievable goals. Such an approach—as opposed to the singular goal of achieving complete pain relief—can help patients regain a sense of balance in their life. While not eliminating the impact of pain, it can diminish how pain impairs our life and enable us to see areas of hope. Periodic review of these goals is important—it ensures we attain them and determines whether they remain a priority.

Define New Physical Boundaries

I would never try to lift a car. The task would be impossible and the attempt likely to injure my body. We all have physical boundaries, activities we will not try. Those living with chronic pain may need to define new boundaries. There will be physical activities likely to increase the intensity of our pain. We need to decide if any of these activities can be eliminated, reduced in frequency, or done differently. Making these decisions consciously and through discussion with family members is an important step. For example:

- Are there outside activities, like digging, that should simply be avoided?

- Should you set a weight limit above which you will not even try to lift?

- Do items in cabinets or closets need to be rearranged to minimize bending or lifting?

- Do you need to agree on a limit to driving distance or time before stopping to assure you are walking and stretching

with appropriate frequency to reduce
aggravating underlying pain?

- Should important family activities
  be scheduled to avoid times of
  greatest fatigue for you?

- Do you need to limit the number of evening
  activities in a given week to avoid cumulative
  fatigue that will be hard to recover from?

- Do vacation plans need to account for your
  heightened sensitivity to heat or cold?

It is hard to accept new physical limitations. Nonetheless, we need to work past the sense of loss, or even embarrassment, and accept realistic limitations. Aging will force us to accept similar limitations. Their premature arrival will be a bitter pill to swallow, but accepting the reality should be more palatable than suffering unnecessary pain.

Address the Emotions Pain Produces

Pain is a provocateur that prefers company. An array of emotions commonly joins its arrival—anger, fear, frustration, and even despair. Patients living with chronic pain must recognize and deal with these emotions. Failure to do so will cause deep-seated problems that are more difficult to resolve.

Anger and frustration often arise from the limitations pain places on physical activity. Sometimes these feelings focus on the sense of injustice ("Why is this happening to me?"). No medicine will provide the answers to the difficult questions raised by a sense of injustice that often accompanies physical suffering. Far too often, patients with chronic pain who wrestle with these issues become sullen and short-tempered, which drives away those most able to help them cope with their struggles. Recognize this potential and deal with it openly. Many have found spiritual or professional counseling very helpful in addressing the difficult emotional issues arising from chronic pain. Thriving in the face of a life of chronic pain requires facing rather than ignoring these issues.

Be Honest About Its Impact on Relationships

Like the extensive reach of our own nervous system, chronic pain touches many areas of our life—including relationships important to us. A patient with chronic pain of unknown origin faces special challenges with key relationships. The inability to determine a definable cause may arouse suspicion in the mind of their physician, while their physician's inability to find the cause and identify a cure may lead the patient to question their physician's competence. When all avenues of investigation yield no cause, family members and employers may question whether the sufferer is really in pain or using pain as an excuse to avoid responsibilities. Patients with chronic pain should recognize these natural reactions and address them openly with complete honesty. It is remarkable how often open communication can dispel suspicion.

Touch can be comforting, even exciting. Fewer things bring warmth like hugging a grandchild. Walking hand in hand with a loved one enriches the most mundane of walks. But touch can escalate discomfort in those living with chronic pain. As a consequence, chronic pain can inhibit one of the most significant ways we engage with those most important to us. They may see us as fragile and withhold physical contact. Conversely, they may not realize the discomfort such contact provokes. Candid discussion about this aspect of our relationships with those in our inner circle is essential to sustain healthy relationships. It is important for romantic partners to know when and how touch is both wanted and enhancing to the relationship.

Chronic pain will influence our mood and reaction to events in life, which will affect those around us. As we learn to navigate the difficult waters of living with chronic pain, acknowledging its effect on those we love and with whom we live life is essential. We must learn how to cope with the experience of pain, and the limitations it causes, in ways that enhance rather than harm these important relationships. This will require communicating to a level many find uncomfortable. Vulnerability in discussing our experience and struggles will enable those in our family, and other important people, to be supportive.

Craig K. Svensson

Recognize Idleness Is an Enemy

For the same reasons pain interferes with sleep, idleness also increases pain. In addition, idleness can give room to brooding, allowing our mind to incubate thoughts of despair about our plight. Brooding can give rise to what clinicians refer to as *pain catastrophizing*. This is a well-described response in some patients with chronic pain, leading to an exaggerated fear of activity or events that may increase pain. It sometimes results in social withdrawal and isolation by those living with chronic pain.

Distraction—drawing one's mind away from a focal point to a new one—is widely embraced as an effective means of reducing the pain experience. Most parents have used this strategy with their children following a painful injury. Sophisticated imaging studies from scientists in Germany and reported in the journal *Current Biology* have demonstrated distraction not only reduces pain perception, but it also alters sensory pain signals in the spinal cord and release of internal pain-relieving chemicals. In other words, there are biological effects of distraction. Studies of this nature indicate keeping our mind and body occupied is an essential strategy for managing chronic pain.

Patients living with pain or disability that limits meaningful physical activity will find a special challenge in guarding against excessive idleness. But it is essential for their well-being to seek and engage in productive activity appropriate to their level of disability. Social engagement is also important. Studies have shown improved mental and physical health in those socially connected to others. There will be times when pain requires us to decline certain social activities. On other occasions, we are better served to push past the pain to remain engaged with people.

I cannot count the number of times pain inclined me to want to withdraw from a planned outing. Being an introvert by nature, I experienced even greater tendency to withdraw from an activity when pain was high. Yet during or after the social engagement, I realized a reduced sense of pain. I enjoyed the engagement, and the distraction minimized my pain. There are times we cannot do something because of pain, but at others times, we must do it for our overall well-being. It is important for us to learn which of these should drive our decision in specific situations.

Those who have withdrawn from social engagements for an extended period out of either necessity or choice will find re-engagement a challenge. Overcoming the barriers to return to involvement with friends and others is essential for our well-being. One does not need to fill the calendar at once with social outings, though. Start with one event at a time. The first step may be as simple as a phone call or online chat to catch up. The next may be a brief outing for coffee or a meal. The level of social engagement will wax and wane in the same manner as our pain. But it is in our best interest not to allow pain to lead to permanent social isolation.

Embrace the Change Pain Has Produced

Living with chronic pain changes things. It does so beyond measure. It is likely we will add certain activities to an inverse bucket list—a do not do list. As discussed before, avoiding activities that unnecessarily increase your pain is wise. Acknowledging these limitations will create a sense of loss. We may dwell on the loss and find ourselves immersed in ongoing sadness. Instead, we can seize the change in our life as an opportunity to explore new avenues and experiences.

Some patients with chronic pain have probed with great depth the nuances of pain—authoring books or blogs they would have never conceived apart from their personal adventure into chronic pain. Melanie Thernstrom, author of the *New York Times* bestseller *The Pain Chronicles*, is a stellar example of one whose personal journey with pain turned her attention to the subject with a perception unlikely to be achieved by those living pain-free. Others have found a voice for suffering through poetry or art. Even more have used their experience to counsel fellow sufferers. Each has enriched the lives of others through refocusing their energy in ways not considered before the limitations chronic pain forced upon them.

Patients whose pain has caused them to abandon one form of physical exercise have sometimes been able to find a new passion through exercises that don't increase their pain. Others have used the physical limitations to devote themselves to new hobbies or other rewarding activities—including intellectual pursuits for which time never seemed available in the past.

Those living with chronic pain are not unique in facing unexpected and undesired changes in their life course. Many ailments produce marked alterations in a patient's life. Other people live with the persistent impact of a traumatic event (such as an assault). For some, a shattered relationship has forever changed their life experience. Others march through life with the persistent pain of the loss of a child or spouse.

The changes these unwanted alterations bring to the life we envisioned can provoke within us a profound sense of loss—or we can embrace the change as an opportunity to seize new adventures. Living with chronic pain challenges us in many ways. We can accept the change or brood over the loss the ailment has forced upon us. Which approach will best enable us to thrive?

Learn from the Revealing Power of Pain

Recently, the stress of renovation on a bridge near my home revealed several construction flaws demanding immediate attention. Failure to address these flaws could result in future disaster. Similarly, stressors in our life—such as pain—can reveal flaws in our character, or our way of thinking and acting, that need attention. If we can accept it, pain will reveal areas of weakness in our life. A proper level of introspection in response to our pain can make us better people.

Walking through life with daily pain revealed, to my shame, my all too frequent judgmental response to people living with invisible illnesses. I far too quickly assumed a negative reason for their absence from work, their sullen affect, and their unwillingness to do marginal physical activity. My journey with pain forced me to recognize my guilt through the fear others would judge me the same way. Pain became something like a mirror for my life—and I was not pleased with all it reflected. Pain gave me the opportunity to address flaws I likely would not have seen without experiencing physical discomfort. I take no joy in living with persistent pain, but I am grateful for the opportunity it afforded me to see myself with better clarity and address more flaws than I'd care to admit.

Living with inescapable distress, such as chronic pain, is one of the greatest challenges of the human experience. But it need not lead to despair. Those who live with unremitting pain can find a path to a fulfilling life—and experience joy nevertheless. Chronic pain will change the course of one's life, but it does not have to lead to a dreary destination. It is in our power to decide the path we will travel.

CHAPTER 5

What to Do When People Say Hurtful Things

"Dr. Svensson plays a power game when you go to his office with a question. While you sit down, he remains standing, always above you. He makes students uncomfortable this way and I think it is intended to discourage them from coming to his office and bothering him with questions." So read a comment among my end-of-semester teaching evaluations during the year my back pain was at its worse. This student did not realize that, due to incessant back pain, I never sat down in my office—whether or not someone else was present. In fact, if the student had looked carefully, they would have seen no chair behind my desk. I had no use for one at this stage in my life. Perhaps my experience is the type Henry Wadsworth Longfellow had in mind when he said, "Every man has his secret sorrows which the world knows not; and often times we call a man cold when he is only sad."

Another episode made me chuckle. As I was walking down the aisle leaving a church service one Sunday, I overheard one elderly woman who was pointing to me say to a visitor, "That's Dr. Svensson. The church has hired him to stand against the wall during church services to provide security." My physical presence would not intimidate even a church mouse. In truth, I stood because it was too painful to sit in the church pew, which seemed designed to provoke discomfort. I cannot count the number of times when standing during a committee meeting or in the aisle during an airplane flight that someone said, "Will you sit down? You are making me nervous standing there!"

The discomfort of others provoked by my standing in the aisle during a flight increased exponentially after September 11, 2001 (the day terrorists destroyed the Twin Towers in New York City). I've had flight attendants tell me it is against federal law to stand in the aisle during a flight (it is not). Shuttle bus drivers at airports have barked at me, saying they can't move until I take a seat although a sign above their head states "passengers must stand behind the yellow line while the bus is moving." There are also straps hanging from overhead bars for standing passengers to hold. Go to an office for an appointment and one of the first things the receptionist will say is, "Please, have a seat." Many find it unacceptable when you decline to do so and resort to rudeness trying to get you to sit rather than stand. On several occasions at my current university, I have needed to leave the public lecture of noted guest speakers in one of our auditoriums because ushers insist I am violating fire code by standing in the back.

Lifting a heavy suitcase provokes increased pain for me, which can last for days after pulling a suitcase off a revolving airport luggage carousel. My thoughtful wife often asks me to stand back to guard our carry-on cases while she retrieves our luggage from the carousel. I could not count the number of times I have received disapproving looks from others who appear appalled that I would let my wife lift a heavy bag while I stand by idle. An experience like this can sullen my mood and make me a less than desirable traveling companion for my wife.

The Challenge of Invisible Illness

Many who suffer with a chronic ailment endure thoughtlessness, rudeness, humor, humiliation, and outright foolishness from those who do not understand what they are experiencing. Their actions and words can be painful and embarrassing—only adding to the negative impact of one's ailment.

Those whose ailments are invisible to others face special challenges. For example, individuals whose invisible ailment allows them to hold a handicapped parking pass will report passersby yelling such things as, "You don't look handicapped to me!" If I search my memory back many years, I would probably find evidence of personal guilt on this one (at least silently expressed). Others struggling with the profound fatigue of progressive disorders have had to bear accusations of being lazy. Judgment from others who visibly assess one's ability or inability adds insult to the experience of chronic illness.

Developing Healthy Responses

It is essential for those with chronic illnesses to develop healthy responses to the inevitable misunderstandings expressed by others. How we handle episodes in which individuals pass judgment on our unseen ailment can impact the joy we experience in life. And yes, I do think the impact on joy is important.

The ability to experience the beauty and wonder of the world, and the richness of the mosaic tapestry of our society's diverse population, markedly influences our outlook on life. How we interpret and respond to life's experiences drives our well-being more than the nature of those experiences themselves. Many of us know individuals whose life circumstances are far from ideal—even downright dismal—yet they exude an infectious joy. We have also known those born with a silver spoon in their mouth who have journeyed on what would appear to be a golden roadway, but they are downright miserable and make those around them join in their misery.

I have also known those who suffer from a chronic illness who live life with a proverbial chip on their shoulder. These individuals are quick to take offense at every thoughtless word or action. The lens through which they see the world and their experiences in it are shaded at every angle by their illness. They seem to thrive in playing the role of a victim. By their response, they bring further misery to their life experience. They have entered a vicious cycle of self-harm, emotionally speaking. Failure to break the cycle leads to further deterioration of their overall health, as well as driving others away.

Speaking with patients who suffer with invisible illness, as well as reading memoirs and blogs of others with such illnesses, reveals that the misunderstanding of others is a common experience for many patients. This misunderstanding, often giving rise to hurtful comments, seems to be among the most painful issues their chronic illness surfaces. How do we deal with the misunderstandings, wrongful judgment, and inconsiderate words of others? How do we avoid the frustration and anger such experiences are prone to provoke within us?

How to Respond to Thoughtless Words or Deeds

First, individuals with an invisible chronic ailment must recognize that a change in this tendency of others is unlikely to occur anytime soon, as cultural change is slow and unpredictable. However, we can control our response when others speak or act in a way that reveals they do not understand what we are experiencing. Focusing on our response instead of the pain produced empowers us to deal with their misunderstanding in a manner that enhances rather than worsens our life experience.

Second, let such experiences remind us of our own guilt. This can prevent us from setting unreasonable expectations for others. How sensitive were we toward those with an invisible illness before we were similarly afflicted? Honesty would cause all of us to admit instances where we have misjudged others.

Third, recognize people will say stupid things. It is an unpleasant fact. I do it quite often myself. On many occasions I have proven the truth of an old adage: "Nothing is more times opened by mistake than the mouth." Nonetheless, stupid comments are not usually intentionally hurtful. Frequently, these thoughtless words reflect an individual's discomfort. They don't know what to say. While the better part of wisdom would suggest silence as the best response, people are uncomfortable with silence. Consequently, they fill the air with words— words that sometimes unintentionally wound others. We can choose to cut them some slack and not quickly assume the motive behind the comment.

Fourth, check our own assumptions. Is the lack of understanding or empathy because we have not communicated our limitations to them? Perhaps their comments reflect a lack of knowledge rather than a lack of sympathy. When I discussed with an individual his obvious irritation with my standing during a business meeting, it was clear he misread the situation. He concluded my standing was an effort to force him to end the meeting so I could leave. When he learned it was to avoid the pain sitting created, he was more than sympathetic to my plight. I learned to comment at the beginning of meetings: "Pardon my standing, but I have a bad back." Interestingly, others have told me that my standing during a meeting has given them the freedom to stand—a liberty they hesitated to exercise until they saw my example. In the opening scenario of this chapter, I could have prevented the student's misunderstanding by being proactive, simply informing the class or individual why I did not join them in sitting when they came to my office.

Fifth, share your feelings of frustration at the misjudgments when they recur. While it is best to ignore most thoughtless comments, if those we do life with do so repeatedly, it is healthy to discuss the issue. Failure to do so may fracture our relationships and give rise to bitterness within us. Flinging a retort like an arrow when they make such comments will only inflame the situation. Instead, find the right time and place to have a candid discussion. It is likely they are unaware of the hurt their comments have caused. We may find the fruit of such a conversation is a new ally in our journey with chronic illness.

Wayne and Sherri Connell are a couple with a special passion for helping those with invisible ailments, as described in their book *"But You LOOK Good."* One outcome of their experience has been to form an organization, the Invisible Disabilities Association, with the explicit purpose to educate people about those who suffer from invisible ailments and encourage those afflicted. They have resources on their website to share with others (www.invisibledisabilities.org).

Sixth, keep your experience in perspective. While not wanting to discount the pain patients with invisible illnesses experience from the hurtful judgments of others, I have found it helpful to reflect on the reality that others have known far deeper pain from the prejudicial judgment heaped on them. When recently reading Dr. Martin Luther King Jr.'s *Stride Toward Freedom*, I realized how petty the slights were that I had experienced from the misunderstanding of others. They bring a twinge of emotional pain, but nothing like the experience of racial and religious prejudice others in our land live with every day. Might such tastes of misplaced judgment from others give us more empathy toward those whose experience is more protracted and ingrained in our society?

Knowing others have endured greater suffering does not take away our pain—but it can help us endure the pain. Not everything that hurts can be fixed. Not every injury can be healed. Some burdens must simply be borne. When I see others enduring greater hardship than me, I am reminded of the resilience of the human spirit. Their ability to stand well in the face of difficulty reminds me I can do the same. It keeps me from turning molehills into mountains.

Finally, recognize that all beauty in this world is imperfect. The most beautiful meadow has some dung in it. The most gorgeous sky has pollutants floating around. Even the most beautiful face is marred—we only need to get close enough to see its flaws. But such imperfection does not negate the beauty of the meadow, sky, or face. Life, including people, can be enjoyed despite the imperfections. We need to decide if we will focus on the imperfections or the beauty.

Everyone has to deal with the messiness of interacting with other people. Those living with an invisible illness may think their experience is unique—

but it is not. Single people can catalogue the insensitive and hurtful comments spoken by married couples. Painful statements made by others frequently wound individuals struggling with infertility. And the list goes on. All of us who journey in human society are occasionally pricked by sharp words spoken by others with insufficient care. We can choose to allow each comment to penetrate deeply. Conversely, we can develop a thick skin and readily deflect such comments, giving them no more time than they deserve. Which path will enable us to live well?

CHAPTER 6

What to Do When You Learn Your Health Will Get Worse

My life unraveled further at about 35,000 feet above the Pacific Ocean. After I spoke at a joint Japanese-American conference, my wife and I enjoyed several days of R&R on Maui. With the love of my life sleeping in the seat beside me on our return flight, I buried my head in a book. The story plot dropped from the forefront of my mind, however, when the pages became blurred. Alternating my eyes revealed a loss of visual acuity in my right eye. Taking my index finger to the farthest right of my peripheral vision, I traced it across my visual field—like an arrow passing across a screen. When my finger entered the field in the middle of my right eye, it disappeared. Probing further, I discovered the extent of vision loss was equivalent to the face of a traditional clock going blank from five to ten o'clock. This was not good. My vision remained stable for the remainder of our travel, so I decided a trip to the emergency room was not necessary when we arrived home late in the evening.

From my university office the next morning, I called the ophthalmology department at our university hospital, explained what occurred, and asked to see an ophthalmologist as soon as possible. The receptionist told me she would schedule me for an eye exam, but the next available appointment was in two months. Patiently explaining I had experienced an acute event of some sort, I expressed that I needed an evaluation as soon as possible. She, just as patiently, told me the earliest appointment was in two months. She responded to my request to speak to her supervisor with a simple refusal, then asked if I wanted the appointment in two months. A call to my internist's office confirmed my need for an evaluation that day, and they promised to contact the opthamology department for me. Near 5:00 p.m., I received a call from the office of a retinal specialist asking if I could come over to the university hospital at once.

No other patients were within sound or sight when I arrived at the ophthalmology waiting area. A young assistant whisked me into an examination room. The retinal specialist joined us before the assistant had time to finish asking her questions. After probing my eye with great care, he made a diagnosis of optic neuritis— an inflammation of the optic nerve. The good news was it would likely resolve and I would recover most of my vision. A course of steroids would speed recovery. Since it was an infrequent diagnosis, he asked if several residents and students could gaze into my retina with their ophthalmoscopes. After these trainees were finished, the retinal specialist stood before me with an intense look suggesting there was something more concerning he had yet to tell me.

"Optic neuritis is often what is called a clinically isolated event," he said. "About 50 percent of people with optic neuritis go on to develop additional neurological symptoms and ultimately are diagnosed with multiple sclerosis. In fact, some neurologists believe most patients with optic neuritis should be treated with a presumptive diagnosis of multiple sclerosis and started on disease-modifying drugs immediately."

I could not have been more stunned if he had hit me between the eyes with the battery end of his ophthalmoscope. I was ready to accept a permanent loss of vision in my right eye. But to learn there was a high chance of a ticking time bomb within me likely to result in further neurological deterioration came out of the blue. Dazed as I walked through the now dark corridors of the ophthalmology department, I returned to my office next door to the hospital. It was fortunate there was no road to cross, as I was oblivious to my physical surroundings as I walked.

My secretary and faculty colleagues had gone home by the time I returned to my office. Standing in the quiet of the department, I was unsure what to do next. Part of me wanted to run home to the comforting arms of my wife. Another part of me said, "I need to know more about what this means before I dump this news on her." She had so patiently walked with me through two chronic ailments. Was our joint journey about to get more complicated? Why this? Why now?

I searched the literature via my computer for studies on the probability of patients like me progressing to multiple sclerosis. The results were discouraging. Chances were high, but there was no way to tell if I would be among those who would manifest other, more disturbing neurological consequences. Only time would tell. Time waiting to see what, if anything, would pop up. Did I dare read more to find out what this diagnosis would mean for my life?

When I got home, my wife's first words made it clear my face betrayed I had an unsettling diagnosis to share. As we talked, the night seemed to grow unusually dark and foreboding. Dinner was unappealing and concentrating on a book afterward no more appealing. Would tomorrow bring the first step to healing or the next decline in my body's function?

More symptoms began a few months after the optic neuritis episode with a complete numbness from the center of my face to behind my left ear. A course of intravenous steroids brought back partial sensation. However, it left a persistent tingling sensation (called paresthesia) from my nose to my left ear. If you've ever received a numbing medication for a dental procedure, you may recall that when the local anesthesia began to wear off, it briefly felt like thousands of needles were pricking the area that was numb moments earlier. This is how the left side of my face feels 24/7/365. It never goes away—ever. Like a perpetually rotating beacon on a lighthouse, this paresthesia has constantly sent its signals across my face for over a decade. Sometimes it exacerbates, but it never disappears. This new symptom upped the suspicion I had MS, but a complex MRI was inconclusive.

A year later, and in a new town, I developed a numbness from my right armpit down to the bottom of my foot. With another course of steroids, the numbness resolved. What remained was my feeling like I had a bad sunburn on the bottom of that foot. It has remained a constant companion since its arrival. This provoked another set of complex MRIs—yielding definitive evidence that I met the criteria for MS.

After almost two years of suspicious symptoms, hearing the pronouncement hit me harder than I expected. As my neurologist delivered his verdict, statistics I read filled my mind. For example, 50 percent of those diagnosed with MS need help walking within five years. He expressed his opinion, and hope, that the age of my diagnosis meant my disease was likely to remain sensory and not result in functional disability. One thing was clear: I should expect a future littered with periodic episodes of further neurological decline. How many, how often, and of what magnitude, no one could tell. The only sure thing was that my course would be downhill.

Living with Medical Uncertainty

Many stories have told of men in trenches in WWI who cracked with anxiety thinking the sounds of the night meant they were about to be pounced on by an unseen enemy. Some became trigger-happy and cut down a trenchmate who had inadvisably chosen to wander into no-man's-land to relieve himself, only to be mistaken as the enemy when returning to his trench. How do I forestall similar anxiety in the face of the uncertain progression of a pathological enemy?

Perhaps no medical assessment is more troubling than those declaring uncertainty of diagnosis or prognosis. When we are living like a watchman in an ancient city tower searching for signs of an emerging enemy, it is easy to perceive that every new or unusual physical abnormality means the enemy has crossed the Rubicon. Anticipatory fear can be as life altering as the ailment itself. How does one live well in the face of the uncertain, but likely, imminent arrival or progression of a pathological enemy?

Some diseases first arrive with symptoms that lead to uncertainty of diagnosis. These include MS, ALS (more commonly known as Lou Gehrig's disease), Parkinson's disease, and several autoimmune diseases (for example, systemic lupus erythematosus, also known as lupus). Patients with these diseases will often report an emerging constellation of symptoms over years before meeting definitive diagnostic criteria. This ambiguity leaves patients waiting for prolonged periods for a clear answer to the cause of their symptoms.

Even more diseases cause patients to face the uncertainty of prognosis. No one can tell with certainty the course the disease will follow in our body. At best, clinicians can slow the progress and give us more time without impairment. At worse, they can put us on a treatment regimen that won't help but whose troubling adverse effects will reduce our quality of life. Decline is certain. Its rate of decrease, not so certain.

Medical uncertainty leaves everyone in discomfort. Clinicians live with this tension daily. A patient may appear to display signs and symptoms consistent with a specific disease, but the presentation varies just enough to leave a measure of doubt. It is probable, but not definitive. In other cases, the symptoms are consistent with several diseases, but the diagnostic criteria are not met for any. In both scenarios, time—associated with additional symptoms developing—will probably provide the answer. Receiving such an assessment is troubling to patients. We want to know what is wrong and may question the competency of a clinician who is unable to provide a definitive answer. This is one of several factors that make clinicians hesitant to communicate their uncertainty to patients.

The tension in this situation escalates when a definitive diagnosis would most likely lead to an intervention to reduce the disease's progression. Will the patient experience harm if treated for a disease they do not really have? Or will they experience harm from failing to get treated for a disease that is present? Writing in the *New England Journal of Medicine,* medical educators have sounded the call to better prepare the physicians of tomorrow to handle this tension of uncertainty.

Being a patient who lives with diagnostic uncertainty presents a different challenge than the one clinicians face. Insight into how patients respond to this uncertainty comes from studies examining the responses of women who have received a suggestive mammogram and are awaiting a breast biopsy and its results. Not surprisingly, such studies show increased stress, anxiety, and depression among patients during the waiting period. On the other hand, delay may enable activation of coping mechanisms before a definitive diagnosis is pronounced. Less is known about the response of patients living through years of diagnostic uncertainty. I recently heard the account of a patient who experienced emerging symptoms for seventeen years before he received a definitive diagnosis of MS. He spoke to the utter frustration of living in a medical quandary for nearly two decades.

Prognostic uncertainty (the inability to predict the future course of a disease) is more common than diagnostic uncertainty. Even for the most straightforward ailments, prognostic precision is low. But it is very low for diseases resulting in a progressive decline of health over years or decades. For example, the course of patients diagnosed with neurodegenerative diseases like MS and Parkinson's disease is variable. It is not possible to accurately predict the course for any given patient. How does one live with such news?

How do patients play the waiting game well when progressive decline is quite certain but its pace and degree unknown?

Take Time to Absorb the Reality

Patients with a chronic disorder have likely lived with diagnostic uncertainty for some time. Now, we must live with the answer as to what is afflicting our body but with no clear answers about the degree and time course of future impairment. The knowledge that we have a serious and potentially debilitating disease changes things. It is unsettling. The usual pace of life often feels like we are living on a racing train. A troubling diagnosis, illness, or loss brings the train to a screeching halt. Everything suddenly becomes still and disorientation sets in. Our routine, expectations, and hopes are dashed in the blink of an eye. Time seems suspended. Dreams are lost in a fog. The news seems to consume everything in our lives. This reality will take time to sink in—for us and for those we love.

Investigators writing in the journal *Epilepsy Research* reported finding over half of patients diagnosed with epilepsy displayed an initial response of fear, depression, or anger. Anxiety and depression are also common among those recently diagnosed with neurodegenerative diseases. Such diagnoses often follow initial symptoms that are suggestive, but further symptoms and diagnostic testing lead to a certain diagnosis. When announced, the diagnosis brings the realization of present and future loss akin to the death of a loved one. The same is true for many chronic diseases.

Patients may well respond with grief. Grief is a natural response to loss. It can also occur when anticipating loss. Substantial research has been conducted on anticipatory grief focusing on the experience of loved ones of those diagnosed with a terminal illness such as cancer. The well-known model of grief by Elisabeth Kubler-Ross arose from her work with cancer patients who were expecting their own death. Less is known about the grieving of those whose anticipated loss is mobility, independence, and fullness of life they now experience.

Unfortunately, too few physicians seem to understand the impact of their diagnostic declarations. Reading about and talking to numerous individuals who have received such diagnoses revealed to me that few received counsel from their clinician about dealing with the emotional aspect of the diagnosis. This is particularly true for those diagnosed with an ailment not expected to take their life, but a disease that will journey with them until their death. I have known patients who live with anger at physicians whose diagnostic pronouncement appeared to them as detached and uncaring. Their physician's apparent callousness has sometimes left them with a sense of abandonment. There is much clinicians can learn from listening to the experiences of such patients.

At the same time, patients need to understand their clinician is facing their own struggle. Anyone who has had to tell another person devastating news understands the inner turmoil of being the bearer of sad tidings. It is distressing to be the one to tell another person they have a degenerative disease. Some specialists have to do this several times a day. The emotional toll on clinicians can be significant. It is not surprising when detachment occurs as a self-protective mechanism. While we might believe they should have handled the situation better, it helps no one for us to harshly judge how they handled the difficult task. Above all, it is harmful to us if we harbor bitterness toward them.

Recognize Sadness Is a Normal Response

A sense of sadness is natural when patients learn that lurking within them is a monster that will, at an unknown rate, cause future functional decline. It is a visceral response to loss. Anticipation of loss can also bring about sadness. It's okay to be sad. It is a normal human reaction. Sadness is one expression of the gravity of the situation. Receiving news about a real or expected loss dashes our hopes and dreams. It changes the expected unfolding of the future. Things will not be as we hoped.

Sadness becomes concerning, however, when it is disproportionate to the loss—in terms of both the magnitude and duration (permanent versus temporary). The depth of sorrow from losing a spouse should be greater than an accident totaling a car one spent many hours restoring. There is no clear line dividing disproportionate from normal sadness, but a skilled clinician or counselor can help patients evaluate their response to difficult life events. If sadness impairs the ability to fulfill responsibilities for a prolonged period (meaning months of impairment), seeking professional or spiritual counsel is advisable.

Engage Those Closest to Us

The advancing pathological enemy within has launched its primary assault on our body. Nonetheless, we must not overlook the impact it is having or will have on those dearest to us. They may share in feelings of anger, fear, and tension from the uncertainty about our joint future. Not wanting to add to our burden, they often will leave these experiences unspoken. But unspoken matters can just as readily impact our valued relationships. Our loved ones need space to deal with this news, in addition to the ongoing ability to engage in open dialogue with us about its impact on their lives. Our empathy to their experience will be as important as their empathy toward ours.

Studies have shown that spouses and partners of those newly diagnosed with a degenerative disease can experience significant distress. The potential need for them to transition to a caregiver can be a troubling realization. Their hopes and dreams for the future have also altered with the diagnosis.

By now, you have probably caught this as a common theme in this book. I emphasize it because I have seen in myself, and others with chronic ailments, the tendency to overlook our malady's impact on others—especially family members. After all, we are the ones with the physical ailment and its accompanying limitations. We are the ones experiencing chronic suffering. But we can't live life closely with others without it impacting their lives.

Among the most important things I wished I learned earlier in my journey was being more attentive to how my ailments impacted others in my family. My ailments had a profound impact on my wife and children, including limiting our ability to travel and my ability to be involved in certain activities with them. I never thought about the fact that my being the only parent standing in the back of the room at a school event would make my teenagers self-conscious. They had to absorb the impact of their dad's last-minute absence at recitals or other important events because I was having a colitis flare-up. Many are the examples of ways my illnesses made their life experience less than I would have hoped. My wife could not count the number of times she has had to explain my absence or inability to do something because of one of my ailments. As patients with chronic illnesses, we need to carefully consider the impact our illness has on others who are close to us.

Avoid the Fruitless Effort to Control What Cannot Be Controlled

Over the years, I have sat through many graduation speeches, and even given a few myself. Speakers often challenge students by telling them such things as, "The future is yours to make!" When I hear such words, I think, "It won't be long before these graduates realize such talk is drivel." Most of the future simply happens to us and is beyond our control. Writing to Albert G. Hodges on April 4, 1864, Abraham Lincoln declared, "I claim not to have controlled events, but confess plainly that events have controlled me." We can control how we respond to the twists and turns that will pop up in our journey through life. But we must discard the notion that we can *control* the future, including the course of our disease. Such notions will lead to frustration when the journey takes us places we do not want to go. Focus instead on how to respond to the inevitable unexpected bumps in the road. Learn how to cope with loss, uncertainty, and the need to be diligent about your health without becoming obsessive. No secret formula exists for doing so, and the tools one deploys will depend on personality, maturity, support system, and spirituality. But patients must find those tools that work for them. Otherwise, we will not live well.

Determine If Preventative
Measures Can Be Taken

Is there anything we can do to stave off this intruder from making headway within our body? For most degenerative diseases, the answer will be no. At least, there are no proven interventions. One can always find recommendations for specific nutritional supplements or dietary alterations that claim to protect us from decline, regardless of the ailment. Truth is, almost none have any reasonable evidence to support their use. Inquirers will also find general health tips directed toward those with an ailment. Such recommendations often reflect common sense and are consistent with generally recommended good health practices. But they are unlikely to alter the course of the disease that afflicts us. Nevertheless, increased attention to healthy practices is advisable when health deterioration is expected due to a degenerative disease.

Learn the Hallmarks Indicating
the Advance of the Disease

At this point, a specialist with expert knowledge of our ailment is most likely providing our care. Frank discussion should occur about how she or he will assess progression over the years to come. Are there symptoms that suggest a more rapid progression? How will the disease affect functional and cognitive abilities? How might these impact professional or personal plans? Should what we know about progression change those plans?

Patients should be cautious about information found on blogs and discussion sites about specific diseases. One can find myriad claims by patients such as, "My disease causes these symptoms." When patients have a degenerative disease, it is easy to attribute all health alterations to the disease. Often, patients' claims of symptoms associated with the disease have not been validated. Patients can forget that those suffering from a chronic illness get other ailments and experience the normal functional declines often associated with aging (see chapter 10 for further discussion on this topic).

Identify What Merits Intervention

Those living with an incurable degenerative disease are prone to two errors. The first is becoming so guarded we see any change in health as a sign of disease progression. The second is ignoring signs meriting attention. It is imperative to learn how to strike the right balance between these two extremes.

Many chronic ailments, even those associated with a progressive decline, wax and wane over time. If there are interventions that can decrease discomfort or reduce potential impairment, patients need to identify benchmarks to indicate when to act. This should include differentiating when self-management is appropriate versus when to see a medical specialist as soon as practical. How one approaches this issue will vary with underlying ailment, options available for intervention, and a patient's own confidence in managing their health.

Watch, but Don't Worry

Worry has to be one of the most unfruitful activities we can undertake. It provides no benefit and can produce negative consequences of the highest order. If especially prone to worry, or if worry becomes an issue, professional or spiritual counseling may be helpful. We all have certain proclivities. Some people are prone to be overly controlling. Others struggle with apathy. If you are inclined to worry about the future, you will benefit by recognizing this tendency and realizing a chronic ailment expected to lead to physical decline will probably lead to worry. Being proactive and seeking wise counsel to help you develop a healthy response to this reality is in your best interest. The diagnosis of a degenerative disease may provoke worry even in those not inclined to brood over the future. If you find yourself ruminating on the what-ifs to the degree that it impairs your ability to enjoy life in the present, or it creates anxiety, seeking professional or spiritual counsel is advisable. Patients should have frank discussions with loved ones about their perceptions of how we are handling this troubling diagnosis.

Uncertainty is unsettling. Unsettling or not, those living with expected health decline at an unknown rate need to keep this uncertainty in perspective. We may not survive the next five-mile car ride we take. Our job could be on the chopping block in the next month. A flu pandemic could strike our neighborhood in any year, decimating the population in short order. The next public event we attend could be the target of a terrorist attack. The simple reality is we always stand on unsteady ground. Life is full of uncertainty. Indeed, life itself is uncertain.

Living with the uncertainty of a disease's progression may feel like holding a ticking time bomb whose countdown timer is inaccessible. We are unsure when it will go off, but we know it will happen. We must learn to deal with the distress such uncertainty can produce. Many have successfully walked this road before us, and we can as well.

CHAPTER 7

How to Deal with Fear About the Changes Disability Will Bring

The blue and red lights in my rearview mirror shook me out of my thoughts. I did not notice the squad car until it was within spitting distance to my rear bumper. How long had he been behind me? A glance at the speedometer showed my SUV was traveling at 66 miles per hour. Surely he was not pulling me over for going one mile over the speed limit? Embarrassed to have not seen him coming sooner and moved out of his way, I pulled off to the shoulder and stopped. He stayed behind me. I could not imagine why he chose me out of the many drivers for a personal visit.

The cool air sent a chill across my face as I lowered my window to speak with the officer. This public servant asserted I was exceeding the speed limit by ten miles per hour. When I expressed my surprise at his claim, he pointed out the speed limit on this stretch of the I-65 north of Indianapolis dropped from 65 to 55 miles per hour three weeks earlier. I fumbled through my glove compartment to uncover the requested registration and proof of insurance. Napkins, CDs, oil change receipts, and papers I did not recognize schemed to lengthen the search time. Instructing me to wait for his return, he walked back to his vehicle with my documents in hand. Feeling like a man kicked when he is down, self-pity arose within me while I awaited the officer's return. The shake of my SUV in response to the eighteen-wheelers roaring by amplified my unsettled feelings.

The officer returned with more papers in hand than he had when he left. He gave me a ticket and instructions of how to make my financial contribution to the local municipality. I thanked the officer for his work keeping us safe and promised to be more careful. I closed my window to the sound of crunching gravel as he sped off to find another citizen to visit. Muttering to myself with frustration at the recent unnoticed decrease in speed limit, I reviewed the ticket to determine how much my bank account would decline. "This is icing on the cake of my day," I thought.

I had not received a ticket in decades, so this traffic violation wasn't a big deal. Yet on this day, it pushed my already tottering emotions on the edge. Unexpected tears swelled into my eyes as I readied to continue my journey home. I didn't need this added hassle while dealing with the inner turmoil from news already sending my mind into a dark descent. The trip to Indy was for a follow-up with my neurologist after an extended MRI—ordered due to further symptoms suggesting emerging MS. During the return trip, my mind focused on the conclusion my neurologist had just pronounced. The expected enemy was no longer at the gate. It had crashed the gate and chipped away at the insulating sheath normally protecting my nerves. Hot spots on my brain and spine visible on the MRI removed any uncertainty. The verdict was in: I had MS.

As I drove back from my appointment, both before and after my unexpected encounter with the man in blue, my mind focused on the logical question—"How does this diagnosis change what I do now?" I especially contemplated the potential long-term consequences for my family, as well as my career as a dean and professor. My mind went to the harshest of outcomes. Will I progress to confinement to a wheelchair? What happens if I can no longer work? What will I do in life if the worst happens? Is my wife destined to become my caretaker?

The Dread of Progressive Decline

Those living with the progressive deterioration of chronic illness often live with the dread of becoming confined—to a wheelchair, a home, a bed, or a machine. A life so restricted is unimaginable. We shudder at the thought. Many declare they would prefer not to live than to live in a world shrunk so small. In desperation, some people take steps not to live in such a state.

After receiving the definitive diagnosis of MS, I found it hard to avoid ruminating on the possibility of a future punctuated with increasing physical disability. My mind went to a former member of my research group who quickly progressed after diagnosis of MS to significant physical limitations. His professional career ended early. I thought of patients with MS whose overwhelming fatigue left them housebound for weeks at a time. Others were wheelchair bound, needing help with the simplest of life activities. A dear friend with chronic fatigue syndrome cut her academic career short and found herself restricted to their home due to a simple lack of energy to do anything. Her life experience became limited to the couch and the bed. Another friend with lupus took on a hermit-like life to avoid the devastating consequences of catching an upper respiratory tract infection from others. Can people thrive when their world has shrunk so small? And can I thrive now with such a possibility on the horizon?

These are questions anyone diagnosed with a degenerative disease must face. Whether it is Parkinson's disease, arthritis, ALS, MS, or some other disease—the fear of this outcome will linger within such patients. It can produce feelings of dread. Dreading the potential of future harm or catastrophe can give rise to a crippling anxiety. Abraham Lincoln is purported to have said, "If I am killed, I can die but once; but to live in constant dread of it, is to die over and over again." In like manner, living with the dread of physical decline is to bear its hardship before it even arrives.

Thriving in Confinement

How do we live with the reality of expected physical decline without giving in to the unsettled feelings of dread? Simply trying to push thoughts of it aside is not a healthy response. Rather, coming to peace with the hard reality will enable one to thrive during the progressive march of physical decline.

The starting point is to recognize that yes, people can thrive in the face of a world far more confined than they now experience. Not that confinement is better. It does not mean there will be no sadness over the loss of mobility, the lack of freedom to spread our wings as far as we please. Nevertheless, we can thrive in the face of a new normal—one very different from our present experience. How can I say this with such confidence? Because others have done so—some with remarkable impact on our world during a time in which their world shrank very small.

Viewed by some as the first English novel, *The Pilgrim's Progress* is an allegory written in 1678. The book has never been out of print since its first roll off the presses. Over the years, this text has been translated into over 200 languages. Remarkably, it was written during the twelve-year confinement of its author, John Bunyan, in the Bedford County jail. Jails in England during the 1600s were not comfortable places. Prison cells were dark, damp, and infested with vermin. Inmates had no access to water or proper means for disposing human waste. No artist appears to have captured the jail that held Bunyan. However, upon visiting this site nearly a century later, the High Sheriff of Bedfordshire was so appalled at the conditions that he devoted his remaining days to penal reform. Despite the conditions, Bunyan produced one of the greatest works of English literature—one still read and studied across the world today. He also wrote his autobiography while confined to this decrepit dungeon.

Helen Keller is a name known to most of us. At nineteen months of age, she contracted an unknown illness, leaving her deaf and blind. At this young age, she entered a world of darkness and silence. The voice of her mother no longer entered her head. The sounds of birds, the pitter-patter of raindrops, and the melodies of childhood songs ceased enriching her world. People, toys, food, clothing, and her own body parts were no longer visible. It was just darkness. Temperature, smell, taste, and touch provided the only stimulation from the external environment. Could one's world shrink any smaller? Amazingly, she overcame these barriers to become the first deaf-blind person to earn a bachelor's degree—something only about 30 percent of the current US adult population has accomplished. Keller published twelve books and traveled the world speaking. Her advocacy on behalf of the deaf and blind brought her great acclaim.

Near to my childhood home in Maryland, Joni Eareckson Tada dove into shallow waters and suffered a life-altering injury leaving her paralyzed from the neck down. She is confined in a body unresponsive to her brain's requests to move. She can't put on her shoes, much less tie the laces. Someone else must do her personal hygiene. She requires around-the-clock help. Despite such physical confinement, and the myriad ailments associated with paralysis, Joni has married, written over fifty books, and is a gifted painter. She founded an organization, Joni and Friends, that has a profound impact on individuals with disabilities. This organization has provided wheelchairs for the disabled across the globe, as well as training for those wishing to help the disabled. They have worked with disability organizations and governments around the world to heighten awareness of the needs of the disabled. Despite her physical limitations, those who encounter her are quick to note that she exudes an infectious joy.

The accounts I've shared are, without doubt, remarkable. Such accomplishments by an unconfined person would be noteworthy. At the same time, they show that it is possible to thrive even when our world shrinks. Most of us find satisfaction with lesser feats than described for these individuals. We should take encouragement from their examples. Our world may shrink as a disease progresses, but it can still be fulfilling. Even when confined to a smaller space, our lives can be impactful.

The Value of Heroic Stories

Stories of heroic feats have been popular throughout human history. Why? Because such narratives inspire us to see what can be, not simply what exists. They encourage us to overcome our own barriers, including personal apathy, and take up the charge to do hard things. Exemplary accounts of the feats of others touch us in a special way.

People facing the barriers of debilitating illness need inspiration. We need narratives to draw us out of self-pity and the inclination to surrender to physical limitations. From time to time, we need encouragement to pull ourselves up by our bootstraps and press on. Stories of those who have accomplished amazing things can provide a clarion call to follow in their steps—or wheelchair tracks, as the case may be. Making such narratives a part of our intellectual diet can provide the nourishment needed to come to grips with our own physical challenges and persevere.

Shortly after receiving the dreaded diagnosis, I had an evening meeting in a community center my church constructed. Awaiting the arrival of others, I peeked into the gym from which shouts of a competitive basketball game arose. As usual, the players were drenched in sweat and breathing heavily. The small crowd robustly cheered the teams as they progressively flowed from one end of the court to the other. But there was no sound of running—for all the players were in wheelchairs. I'm certain each cruised down the court faster than I could run. Smiling as I turned to head to my meeting, I thought, "I can do this."

Craig K. Svensson

Coming to Grips with the Prognosis

To deal with the prognosis that our physical abilities may decline prematurely, we must first recognize this reality need not be devastating. Dramatically life altering? Without doubt. Life will be different. Even so, life can be rich. We can know joy amid physical decline and make a difference in the lives of others. We likely won't change things on a global scale—for few ever do. But we can impact the corner of the world in which we live.

On the morning of my twenty-fifth birthday, I received an unexpected call from an elderly couple I had never met. As a single man who recently arrived in town, I did not know many people. A call shortly after the crack of dawn was unusual. This couple called before I left for the university to sing happy birthday. No one would urge them to record a CD of themselves, but their song was sincere. I learned they were an aging couple in my church whose physical limitations confined their world, but not their hearts for other people. Part of their calling in life became telephoning members of our church to wish them a happy birthday. Apart from a call from my parents, it was the only birthday wish I received the entire day. As you might suspect, it lightened my heart and gave me a warm feeling as I began my day.

This couple found a simple way to make a difference in the lives of others. Being housebound did not shrink their world as much as others thought. Their life was different, but it remained meaningful. True, they received no national awards for their work. Perhaps this recounting is the only public acknowledgment of their

118

deeds. I don't even recall their names. Regardless, they made a difference in the world in which they lived. Can any of us expect to do more than this? Is making such an impact fulfilling?

In reality, all who live to an age approaching a century will experience a decline in body functions. All of us will find physical activities we cannot do or do as well. Losing physical ability will be the plight of every man and woman who lives long enough. Some may face the physical limitations earlier, or to a greater degree, through disease or injury. But we are all on the road to physical decline. If we perceive our value to be in our physical abilities, we will probably face a future of despondency. The elements of our being that really matter are not tied to physical ability.

This is not to deny the hardship physical limitations create. The impact on one's life can be profound. Loss of mobility comes at a high personal cost. Things that once brought joy and fulfillment have flowed down the drain of disability. Those living with serious physical limitations merit our empathy and help.

Finding Help

At the same time, people with a prognosis including the *potential* for future physical limitations should not dwell on this possibility. We can become so concerned about the future that we fail to experience the present to its fullest. If we find ourselves in a perpetual cycle of worry over the potential future, we should seek spiritual or professional counsel. A conversation with one who has traveled down the same road may well empower us to do the same.

Some people find help in support groups focused on specific diseases. Apart from support groups in the context of economic development in emerging economies and those focused on mental health issues, little research exists on the effectiveness of such groups. Their impact on health outcomes remains unknown. Nonetheless, it makes sense that meeting with people whose disease has progressed further can provide insight and a greater understanding of the resources available to assist patients. Some patients have found such groups to be one way to allay their fears of the future. The Mayo Clinic has produced a helpful guide for patients considering a support group (www.mayoclinic.org/healthy-lifestyle/stress-management/in-depth/support-groups/art-20044655). The nature of these groups varies and aligns with the participants' personalities. Some take on an aura of despondency, while others provide an atmosphere of encouragement. Writing for the New Jersey Self-Help Group Clearing House, Merrill Altberg has written a helpful piece on this entitled "Ways to Prevent Your Group from Becoming a 'Pity Party'" (www.njgroups.org/532-2/). Finding the right group is important. One that drags you down should be removed from your calendar.

It is also helpful to realize the incredible growth in technical assist devices expanding the abilities of those with physical disabilities. Working on a university campus with a commitment to technological innovation enables me to learn of exciting areas under development. Some of our brightest young minds have dedicated themselves to deploying advances in technology to assist those whose physical abilities are limited by disease or injury. I take great encouragement in how many young people are committed to using their intellect and energy to improve the plight of those in need. Suffice it to say, the world of helpful devices on the horizon promises to enable those facing future disability to more easily overcome barriers than those living with disability today. This should be reason enough to caution us against forecasting our future experience should our world shrink through physical limitations.

Planning for the Future

It is wise to consider ways we might change things in our life to accommodate future disability. For example, I have friends who built a new home with doorways, hallways, and a bathroom able to accommodate a wheelchair. The wife was and remains ambulatory, but her ailment will likely lead to her needing a wheelchair. It made sense for them to consider this when investing in building a new home. If one lives in a multistory home, considering a move to a single level may make sense if physical limitations are possible in the near future. It has surprised me how many people do not consider the likelihood of physical decline when building a retirement home. Such decline is inevitable if they live long enough.

People who are highly active are wise to consider less strenuous activities that will still provide fulfillment for their leisure time. Exploring new hobbies makes sense if expected physical decline will require you to set aside your primary recreational activities. Being prepared to transition to different pursuits will decrease the sense of loss if such limitations occur. As noted earlier, such decline is inevitable with age anyway. Many do not age well because they do not prepare for such changes. Some of us are forced to think about this sooner and may be better prepared as a result.

Some patients diagnosed with degenerative diseases have physically demanding jobs. It may make sense to consider alternative careers—and even seek out essential education to prepare for them—if possible decline will impair your ability to fulfill your current duties. Part of my motivation for preparing for life as a writer was recognizing I may not be able to continue my academic career as long as planned. I am not ready to hand in my resignation at the university, but I know what I will do with my time if it becomes necessary. If decline does not cut my career short, I will be content expanding my writing time after retirement.

Planning is prudent. Brooding is unhealthy. It is important to know the difference between the two. Patients should evaluate their insurance policies. Discussion with a financial planner, including the what-if scenarios, is wise. Think through potential career options. Discuss with loved ones how to address housing changes if or when things deteriorate physically.

But avoid dwelling on the worst-case scenario. For a variety of reasons, it may never happen.

Shortly after the first of each year, I update a document I created many years ago entitled "In the event of my death." It contains all the relevant information someone would need after I die: life insurance policy information, banks account numbers and locations, retirement fund accounts and contacts, attorney for my will, etc. Each year I review the document, make needed changes, and provide a copy to my wife and daughter (the executor of our estate). I don't give it another thought until after the first of the next year. I have planned for the inevitable, but it does not unnecessarily occupy my thoughts and energy.

In the same way, we should not ignore a likely future of disability. Take time to think about and discuss key issues with the important people in your life. If specific action will ease the potential transition, take the needed steps to put a plan in place. Create a time frame to periodically revisit and revise your plan. This will help you strike the balance of proper planning while avoiding obsessing over the future.

Coming to grips with potential limitations in the future means they no longer instill fear within us nor leave us without a sense of control in our lives. While it may be something just over the horizon, we set it aside for now. Wisdom is found in the adage, "We'll cross that bridge when we come to it." Others have done so successfully. When the time comes, we too can cross over into a smaller world and continue to thrive.

CHAPTER 8

How to Choose the Best Course When All Your Options Have Risk

My left hand gripped a syringe filled with a clear solution. Like early morning dew on a spider's web, a tiny drop of fluid dangled from the edge of the needle tip—the residual of my effort to expel air bubbles. Staring at the needle, I grimaced knowing what was to follow: a quick thrust into my thigh and then pressing the plunger. Next came the burning, like a sting from a bat-sized bee. I gritted my teeth to prevent groaning at the torment. Every day of every week of every month of every year for five years I performed this ritual. Should I continue to bow before this deliverer promising delayed disability? Is it worth it? Is this medicine bringing enough benefit to merit bearing this discomfort?

The alternative treatments for MS at the time were less attractive. One required just a weekly injection but left in its wake flu-like symptoms for up to forty-eight hours. Feeling like I have the flu for one to two days every week? No thanks. Two other medications caused a low incidence of a rare viral infection in the brain. Not likely to happen, but if it did, the outcome would be devastating. None of the options would reduce my current symptoms. At best, they slowed descent to disability. If I took none of the medications, well, the disease would just chew away at my nerves at a pace of its choosing. Some options, huh?

Many patients with a progressive chronic ailment face difficult decisions. They are caught between options, each having the potential for bad consequences. The choice often centers on medical treatment possibly slowing disease progression but known to cause significant adverse effects. Often referred to as disease-modifying agents, drugs are available for treatment of arthritis, Crohn's disease, MS, and other disorders believed to be autoimmune in origin. Some agents may shorten the length of a relapse, while others slow progression over the long-term. Many are marginally effective. All carry substantial risk of adverse effects, ranging from simple discomfort to life-threatening brain infections. How do we decide if a therapy is worth the risk? What is the risk of doing nothing?

Other patients face the choice of surgical interventions, which may or may not improve their condition. The anesthesia alone puts them at risk, but the intervention itself could be harmful. Scar tissue could cause a new source of persistent pain, or even restrict mobility. An inadvertent nick of a nearby blood vessel or nerve during surgery could be disastrous. What if you go through the agony of recovery—with lost days of work and ridiculous medical bills—but are no better in the end? What if you are harmed rather than helped?

The Trap of Decisional Conflict

These decisions can be agonizing for patients and their families. Sometimes we find ourselves trapped in what psychologists call *decisional conflict*, which is the tension caused by uncertainty about what we should do when facing potential loss, harm, or regret from the decision. Researchers have found that the presence of decisional conflict can delay treatment, result in poor adherence to therapy, produce long-term regret over decisions made, and even provoke conflict between physicians and patients. Those of us living with chronic ailments will probably face this scenario many times over the course of our diseases, so it is essential to develop strategies for deciding about medical interventions.

There are three key contributors to the tension arising in a state of decisional conflict. First is a gap in information. We simply don't have sufficient knowledge to make an informed decision. Second is a lack of understanding of how personal values drive medical decisions. What is most important to us as patients, and do those values differ from those of our physicians? Third is an unsupportive environment. Too often we feel pressure from family or others to choose one specific option. Understanding these factors helps us see our way to a strategy of sound decision-making.

Take Time When Making Difficult Decisions

Decisions that may help long term but provide no benefit in the near term should not be made quickly. Even when benefit is gained soon, rarely do we have to make a decision when we are first presented with treatment options. We are unlikely to make our best decisions immediately upon receiving difficult news. Researchers who study decision-making refer to the state of being when patients are first presented with a decisional dilemma as a hot state. Emotions run high. The information communicated and its implications seem overwhelming. Clarity of thinking is often elusive at this stage.

Several years ago, I developed a persistent rapid and irregular heart rate. When the EKG technician in the cardiologist's office hooked me up to her machine, she looked at me with concern and asked, "Are you okay?" Not what you want someone to ask as they view your EKG! The cardiologist soon entered and informed me I was in atrial flutter—a persistent irregular and rapid rhythm. He listed all the adverse events I was at high risk for, such as stroke, heart failure, and lethal arrhythmia. He laid out a course of action to reduce my risk of stroke, followed by a path to getting my heart back into a normal rhythm. A nurse who managed patients on anticoagulants (sometimes called blood thinners) then entered, providing detailed instructions about the drug and the serious risks it presented. Being in atrial flutter put me at risk for several bad consequences. The treatment also put me at serious risk for adverse events, including bleeding into the brain. Doing nothing could cause a life-altering (or life-ending) event. Yet the same was true with the treatment.

I used to manage the anticoagulant therapy of such patients myself and understood all the facts. I taught this stuff in the classroom for years. But when the diagnosis and risk arrived at my doorstep, it seemed overwhelming. A friend who was in the office reception area waiting for his own appointment as I departed told me later I looked to be in a daze. I was in a hot state and not in the best position to make important decisions. When I later sat with my wife to tell her about my visit, I remembered little apart from the potential adverse consequences.

Patients are better served by a cooling period to allow the trauma of the news and the impact of the decision to sink in. We should take the time to gather and consider as much information as we need to decide with confidence. A decision without confidence is prone to lead to living with regret, especially if a poor outcome arises from the choice.

Clarifying Values in Medical Decisions

We should also recognize medical decisions involve values, not just data from clinical studies. Whether they recognize it, clinicians bring their own biases (often rooted in their personal values) into their recommendations for patients. Some are conservative in their approach to treatments, which may be congruent with some patients and differ from others. Other clinicians take an aggressive approach, which suits many of their patients well but not others. If these values go unrecognized as an important part of decision-making, decisional conflict is likely to arise.

Research indicates that sociocultural factors play an important role in patient decisions about treatment for chronic diseases. But evaluating options in the context of personal values can be challenging. A careful review of numerous studies by researchers found that decision aids, which help patients think through options, can be an effective tool in promoting decisions consistent with patient values. Patients should ask their specialist if they provide such a tool. If not, The Ottawa Hospital Research Institute has a helpful online compendium of available patient decision aids for many diseases (https://decisionaid.ohri.ca/azlist.html).

Avoiding Pressure from Others

Many of us can recall an occasion in our childhood where we had to choose for our classmates. As the teacher awaited our decision, our classmates jumped up and down, shouting out what they wanted us to choose. The pressure provoked by the myriad voices created a heightened tension surrounding the decision, which was about something inconsequential in the grand scheme of things. But the likelihood of making a poor choice for the wrong reason was high because of the cacophony of voices in the room. In the same way, family and others pressing us about medical choices does not help us make a decision with the confidence we made the best choice. We need to make important medical decisions free of unnecessary pressure. This means giving ourselves the time and space needed for meaningful reflection.

Making Difficult Choices

How we make difficult medical decisions will depend on our perspective of personal medical care. Do we prefer to trust a sage to guide us down the right path? Allowing a trusted clinician's expressed opinion to direct our care is a viable option. Studies show a large portion of patients prefer to delegate decision-making about treating health conditions to their physicians. If we have confidence in their judgment and don't want to concern ourselves with the nuances behind the decision, then by all means, we should embrace their recommendation and move forward. It is the easiest path and one a significant proportion of patients prefer. Autonomy includes the freedom to delegate a decision to others.

In this case, finding the right clinician to trust is the key decision. There are many paths to choosing the right specialist—one engendering trust and in whose expertise we have confidence. Some will make such decisions based on the advice of trusted friends. Others will choose based on location—for example, a specialist in an academic medical center versus a community practitioner. Many will place their confidence in whatever specialist their primary care provider recommends. Evidence does not support the notion one path will lead to a better outcome compared to other paths.

For other patients, ownership of such an important decision is a priority. They want to control what happens to them in the fullest sense. These patients want the learned opinion of experts, but they also want to control the steering wheel throughout their journey. Because those of us living with chronic illness often make important medical decisions, we are well served to think carefully about how such decisions are made. I highly recommend *Your Medical Mind: How to Decide What Is Right for You* by Drs. Jerome Groopman and Pamela Hartzband (Penguin Books, 2012). I know of no better resource for helping patients develop a sound strategy to think through challenging medical decisions.

Studies into how patients, and their providers, make decisions reveal key steps when facing medical dilemmas:

Avoid decisions based on anecdotal information. Stories are powerful. Those from people we know and respect are especially potent. This is why advertisers often seek celebrities to give testimonials about the value of their product. Their stories seem to grip our heart with a strength the rational mind struggles to overcome. Yet one person's story may be a complete anomaly—180 degrees opposite of what the vast majority experience and unlikely to represent the results we will see.

Anecdotal information is not irrelevant. Nonetheless, the risk of choosing based on an outlier's experience is high, because an outlier is just that—a response unlikely to happen again. We may have encountered someone whose life was spared because they were thrown from a vehicle engulfed in flames after a collision—a vehicle in which they would have been trapped if wearing their seat belt. This unique situation does not mean we are safer if we drive without fastening our seat belt. Much evidence shows we are far more likely to avoid harm by wearing a seat belt than we are to experience harm from doing so. Anecdotal information, such as testimonials, should be placed in context. We need to determine if the anecdotal report represents a common or rare experience.

Sometimes anecdotes give hope. For example, the rare individual whose cancer responded to the last-ditch effort with an experimental drug. Their experience suggests, though the likelihood may be small, you too could benefit from the therapy. Can this hope sustain you through the agony the treatment will provoke? Is the potential you could also be an outlier worth knowing? Does it help you make an informed decision? The answer is probably yes to each of these questions.

Other times anecdotes cause unnecessary fear. In my mind, I can still see the first patient I encountered with a rare severe skin reaction to a drug that caused her skin to slough off her body like a snake shedding its skin. It was almost forty years ago, but the image remains in my memory. The chance of my having the same reaction to this drug is one in a million. I know this well. Such reactions were the focus of my research for years. Even knowing these facts, I am not sure I could take that same drug if it was the best choice for an ailment for me. Irrational thinking? Certainly. But images are incredibly powerful. Overcoming them with facts is hard.

Hence, anecdotal information may be a part, but should not be the sole source, of information for decision-making. My Aunt Ida's experience with a treatment may represent a rare response, or it may be the norm. I need more information to determine which is true. Once I assess this, I will know how to apply what I've learned from Aunt Ida's experience.

Get specific information on the likelihood of outcomes, both good and bad. Today's patients are empowered with information unknown to those who traveled a similar road in previous generations. At times, however, the sheer volume of information can make us feel we are trying to drink from a wide open fire hydrant. Go to the search engine of your choice, type a keyword or two, and bingo—you have more information than you could ever hope to digest. There are too many options on the menu. What is important to learn as we seek information about our options?

When we find ourselves between a rock and a hard place, what we need to know is the possible outcomes of our options and how likely it is we will experience these outcomes. Specifically, we need to know the:

- **Consequences of taking no therapy.**
  Determine how likely it is bad things will
  happen if we take no therapy. Our decision
  may differ if it is almost certain bad things
  will happen versus a 10 percent likelihood.
  How soon are these outcomes to appear?
  Are they months, years, or decades away?

- **Benefits of therapy.** Determine how likely it
  is the therapy will prevent these bad disease
  outcomes. Is the therapy effective in most
  patients or just a few? Are there factors that
  make it more or less likely the therapy will
  work in patients? Do I fit into a category less
  or more likely to experience an outcome?

- **Risks associated with the therapy.**
  Determine the adverse effects of the therapy
  and how likely they are to occur. Do most
  patients have some level of adverse effects or
  just a few? Can I do anything to reduce the
  risk of adverse effects? Are these reversible?

Unfortunately, important information about adverse
effects is difficult to find. Clinical studies reporting 25
percent of patients experience nausea is not very helpful.
What do they mean by nausea? A huge difference exists
between feeling queasy for an hour after taking a drug
versus the hanging-over-the-toilet-for-two-hours kind
of nausea. Knowing both the likelihood of a negative

outcome and the magnitude of its impact on our life are important for making an informed decision. Here is a place where adding anecdotal information from multiple sources to the raw numbers about risk can be helpful. The numbers will tell us the likelihood of the adverse effect occurring, while anecdotes provide a portrait of the patient experience when it occurs.

Patient discussion boards or blogs are sources of unfiltered anecdotes. We need to be cautious about drawing conclusions from such anecdotes since patients will often attribute symptoms to a drug just because they occur while taking the drug. These symptoms may be coincidental and not caused by the therapy. This possibility complicates knowing what to think about patient-reported experiences. It is advisable to seek an assessment of such anecdotal reports from our specialist. We can ask, "I've read some patients who claim to have experienced this effect from the therapy. Have you had patients with similar adverse effects?"

Determine if physician recommendations represent their preference or true difference in outcomes. It is unrealistic to think recommendations from physicians, or even panels of experts, would be free from bias. Ample evidence in research literature shows this to be an unreasonable expectation. Speak to a urological surgeon and he will most likely recommend surgery for prostate cancer. Get advice from a radiologist for the same patient and she will probably recommend radiation. Yet the collective studies done to date don't show better outcomes for one treatment option for prostate cancer over the other. Studies also show geographical biases in treatment preferences for many diseases (including hypertension and thyroid cancer) among clinicians. It is surprising how often treatment guidelines differ between Europe and the United States. Often this difference means no clear evidence is available to select one treatment over the other. As a patient trying to choose, it is important to know if this is the case.

If experts can't agree, how are we supposed to decide which is best? Actually, this scenario is empowering for patients. If there is no clear clinical evidence to support one option over the other, it leaves us with the freedom to choose based on our preference. If data shows surgery is better than drug therapy, I may choose surgery even if I hate the idea of going under the knife. In other words, I may hold my nose and swallow the option best supported by studies. But if studies show no benefit of one option over the other, I can choose the one best suited to my values and general approach to life.

How do we uncover whether preference is driving a recommendation our clinician has made? Begin by asking for the basis for their recommendation. Ask them to explain why they feel that option is the best choice. Seeking a second opinion can also be revealing—as disagreement among recommendations often reveals preference is driving their recommendations. Then use the power of the internet to inform you. There are many useful sources where patients can find information about the evidence behind treatment options. These include the National Institutes of Health, the American College of Physicians, disease-focused societies (for example, the Arthritis Foundation), and patient advocacy groups. The National Institute for Health and Care Excellence, based in the United Kingdom, has a website (www.nice.org.uk) that provides guidance for treating many chronic ailments and is accessible for the nonexpert.

As patients, the preference of others should not drive our choices. When the outcome between choices is ambiguous, clinicians should respect and support patient preferences—setting aside their personal inclinations. We need to push back against a clinician who tries to press us in a certain direction despite the lack of evidence to support the clinician's preference. We want to know and understand the reason behind their preference. Nonetheless, if we reluctantly accept a path charted by our physician's preference, we are likely to live with regret if the outcome is negative.

Pushing back against a recommended treatment plan involves conversations most of us find difficult. It can be intimidating to talk with a specialist whose expertise far surpasses your knowledge in the area. When you feel you are being pressed into an option you are not comfortable with, it is best to hit the pause button. "I am going to need to give this some thought" is an appropriate response. This will give you time to think things through, perhaps even discuss the option with your family, and formulate your response. Importantly, make sure you communicate why you are uncomfortable with the recommended path. If you feel intimidated having such conversations, consider bringing a loved one with you for support at the follow-up consultation.

Clarify and communicate your own values. It is imperative to consider things most important to us that may be affected by the choice. This includes our personal tolerance for risk, which will vary among patients. Some patients are by nature aggressively proactive. They need to know they are doing everything within their power to fight the disease. They can live with an adverse consequence of therapy, as long as they know they did everything they could. Others would find it difficult to live with the consequences of a serious adverse event from a drug they took, while they could accept the outcome of disease progression in the face of no treatment. We need to know where we stand on such matters and communicate this to our healthcare providers.

Personalize the potential outcomes of your various choices. A drug causing a dry mouth may create a real problem for an elementary school teacher who needs to speak all day, but less so for a computer programmer who works in isolation. In deciding among therapeutic options, we need to think through the impact of various outcomes in the context of our life—at work, home, and recreation.

Thinking through the change in our life likely to occur if we experience a bad outcome helps us understand the risk we are considering. This should include the emotional impact. Sometimes, treatment presents us with a significant short-term risk. Once the intervention (for example, surgery) has passed, however, the risk is no longer a threat. On the other hand, doing nothing may leave us with a perpetual low risk. What will be the emotional impact on us in these two scenarios? One person may be more comfortable with a higher short-term risk than the perpetual emotional drain of a long-term risk.

Share your thinking with someone you trust. As an educator, I have always found the process of teaching to add clarity to my thinking. Communicating a reasoned assessment of a subject with someone else often helps me identify gaps in my thinking and see things in context. Another person can see errors in thinking I miss. For the same reason, physicians will often present difficult cases to colleagues—sometimes one on one, at others times in weekly conferences of physician groups devoted to this purpose. Patients facing difficult choices can benefit from a similar approach.

Finding the right person is important. It is most helpful if the person understands our values and is a good listener. Our goal in sharing our thinking with another is not to get either their opinion or affirmation. Rather, it is to seek help in identifying potential blind spots or irrational lines of thinking. They may raise questions we have not considered.

In seeking the right confidant, consider those you know who show wisdom in their decision-making. An individual with a history of knee-jerk reactions to circumstances is not a good option. In contrast, one who has navigated difficult circumstances well is an attractive choice. It must also be someone with whom we feel comfortable revealing our innermost concerns. Importantly, we must trust them to keep the discussion confidential. We should communicate our aim from the outset, explicitly telling them we want their help in assessing our decision-making process, not advising us on the actual outcome. This frees the confidant from feeling responsible for our ultimate choice.

We want to make a decision with confidence—a sense of assurance we have weighed the pros and cons in the context of our lives with sufficient care. The right person will help us with the process rather than try to direct us to a destination of their choice.

Determine what might cause you to change your mind. The decision to undergo surgery must reach a point of no return—a time at which you will or will not undergo surgery. At this point, turning back is not an option. In contrast, chronic therapy need continue only for as long as it is in our best interest. The right choice for the moment may not remain so for the rest of our lives. In deciding to undergo a therapy with meaningful risk, it is worth thinking through in advance what might change our mind on the matter.

While I first decided on a therapy requiring a daily injection (a selection made because it had the best evidence of slowing progression to disability in MS patients), an adverse event and a new therapy on the market changed my choice. Before beginning the injections, I had determined that an oral therapy introduced to the market with at least equal benefits and a similar safety profile would be reason to switch. So I evaluated each new therapy introduced to the market, and when I found one that met these criteria became available several years ago, I decided to change therapy.

Advances in science are continually providing clinicians access to new tools to assess therapy effectiveness and risk. For example, genetic tests are now available to provide guidance for risks of adverse effects of certain drugs and the likelihood they will be effective in specific patients. As more tests of this nature become available, it is reasonable to reassess therapeutic decisions previously made. Furthermore, experience with approved therapy over time may provide new insight into who should and should not receive specific therapies. Persisting with a therapy may no longer make sense in light of such developments.

Does this leave us in a perpetual state of reassessing decisions? In some sense, yes. Medical science advances too rapidly to ignore developments important for our health. This does not mean we need to be on the perpetual lookout for such developments ourselves. While some patients seem to thrive on keeping up with the latest gains in knowledge about their disease, others will not want to bother with information that is not actionable. In the latter case, we can communicate with our specialist the kind of development we would like to know about. We may periodically inquire, "Are there any new therapies you think I should consider?"

Recognize even the best choice may result in a bad outcome. Several years ago, I entered a hospital for a procedure to treat a persistent arrhythmia no longer controlled by drug therapy (I alluded to this earlier in the chapter). I chose a cardiologist over an hour from our home because he was one of the best in the country. He developed the procedure and used it more than any other cardiologist. While I was in a drug-induced dreamland, he spent six hours probing my heart—mapping electrical signals and zapping appropriate areas to prevent strays. Near the end of the six-hour procedure, he inadvertently and unknowingly poked a hole in the upper chamber of my heart. He withdrew his catheters and nurses wheeled me to recovery.

After taking a brief break, this cardiologist began a multihour procedure on another patient. Meanwhile, with each beat of my heart, blood was seeping into the surrounding protective sac around my heart. Eventually, enough blood collected in my pericardial sac to prevent the normal filling of my heart (a condition known as cardiac tamponade). I slid into cardiogenic shock and required an emergency procedure to keep me from needing a grave before day's end. An anticipated overnight hospital stay turned into several days, followed by an emergency readmission after discharge to deal with further unexpected complications.

Leaving the arrhythmia untreated would put me at risk and in great discomfort. The intervention to treat it carried with it a small risk of serious consequences—including death. Either choice left me at risk for a bad outcome. In the end, I came within minutes from experiencing the worst of outcomes. Yet I developed no regret over my decision, despite an unexpected hospital stay and lengthy recovery. I took time to decide what to do—researching options, risks, and potential specialists. I recognized that even in the best of hands, misadventures happen. I could live with this knowledge. But I don't think I could have lived with a decision I felt pressured into. This conviction is common among patients who are able to avoid the tension that decisional conflict creates. By getting the right information, choosing options consistent with their values, and deciding without pressure, they can avoid the sting of regret.

Patients often face the dilemma of less than ideal choices. Each road could lead to a bad end. Unless an emergency, such decisions should be made with great care to avoid living with buyer's remorse. A thoughtful approach will enable us to face decisions with confidence and bear the outcome without regret.

CHAPTER 9

Should You Tell Others About Your Illness?

He entered my hospital room with uplifted brows, wide-open eyes, and a hesitant step. "I never expected to see you here in this condition, Dean Svensson," he stammered in surprise. As a third-year student in our Doctor of Pharmacy program, our local hospital provided part-time employment for him to take medication histories of new patients. He was experienced in meeting and interviewing patients unknown to him, so encountering someone he knew was unexpected.

I was discharged from a medical center in Indianapolis two days earlier (a premature discharge as it turns out) after a medical error during a cardiac procedure jeopardized my life (described in the last chapter). Hours before the student pharmacist entered my room, my wife rushed me to this local hospital because I was gasping for breath. Emergency room staff initially assumed it was a recurrence of cardiac tamponade. The cause of my breathlessness turned out to be unexplainable pleural effusions filling the sac around my lungs with fluid. The usual treatment is to drain the fluid to restore normal filling of the lungs with air. In my case, physicians could not perform this procedure until the effect of an anticoagulant in my body wore off. So, they admitted me for careful observation and oxygen. This left me gasping for breath for the next eighteen hours.

As this student pharmacist asked about my medications, I faced the dilemma of revealing a secret kept from everyone in the university, apart from my personal assistant. One of my current medications gained FDA approval for treating MS and nothing else. Stating this drug as part of my regimen would reveal my diagnosis. There were no concerns about the student's ability to keep the information confidential. However, on the advice of a neurologist, I kept the circle of those who knew I suffered with MS small. I had not arrived at the hospital planning to reveal this to anyone in my college, let alone a student.

Those of us who struggle with chronic ailments face the dilemma of whether we should reveal our ailment, to whom, and when. This is especially true for those whose disease will probably cause disability that may affect our cognitive abilities or mobility. Professional opportunities may be impacted if people have concerns about our ability to fulfill job duties in the future. Potential life partners may worry about the impact our potential disability will have on their life experience. Lenders may question our true future income if an evolving disability changes our likelihood of continued employment. In addition, most of us don't want to be seen by others through the lens of an illness, for it does not define us.

My first neurologist raised the need for me to think about whom to tell. Not long after further symptoms suggested my episode of optic neuritis was probably the harbinger of emerging MS, I accepted a position at another institution. When I connected with the neurologist by email to tell him of my impending move, and to thank him for his care, he suggested we get together for coffee and a farewell chat. I talked with him about people I knew at the medical center in Indianapolis I could connect with for suggestions of a neurologist if he did not know of one to recommend. With my new position, he pointed out, I would be a public figure in the academic and healthcare community. The prestige of the position and university would also provide visibility and experience likely to lead to further career advancement opportunities—if I so desired. He then challenged me to think about the wisdom of revealing any evidence that I might have MS to people who did not need to know. As we talked it through, I came to better realize why he had been slow (in my perception) to stamp the definitive label of MS on me. I embraced his wise counsel, keeping the circle of those who knew to a small and trusted group of individuals. Writing this book involved a conscious decision to abandon the strategy at this point in my life.

Patients who have developed an undefined ailment resulting in a progressive constellation of symptoms, or are newly diagnosed with a disease likely to lead to a troubling future, should consider with care whom to tell and when. Knowledge of important health information can be used to our advantage, but it can also be misused. It is not something to convey lightly. We may need to engage others in helping us think through this issue. A special word of caution is needed in our era of prolific communication via social media.

There is an old story of a prominent Englishman who was visited on his deathbed by a man who had repeatedly slandered him. This repentant antagonist told the dying man he wanted to take his words back. The dying man handed this antagonist a pillow and asked him to tear open one end and release the feather contents out the window into the blustery wind. Though it was a strange request, he complied. Having accomplished the deed, he returned to the dying man's bedside—who then asked the slanderer to go retrieve all the feathers. "Why, the task is impossible," exclaimed the slanderer. "Yes," declared the dying man, "and you can no more rescind your slanderous words." In a similar manner, information released on the internet sustains a life of its own with no efficient means of death. Be cautious about revealing health information to the worldwide web! The wisdom of Solomon is relevant here: "the one who has understanding holds their tongue."

Whom to Tell

The decision of whom to tell will be partially based on the implications, both near and long-term, of our ailment. Our values and personality will also influence this decision. In considering the circle of those we plan to inform, we should ask, "If I were in the other person's shoes, would I feel it important that I know about this ailment?" There are consequences from telling people. But there are also potential consequences of not telling people. Our relationship with others may be harmed if they find out about our disease from others. There is value in asking oneself, "Why would I want this person to know of my ailment?" Is there a sense they have a right to know because of how it will affect them? Do you want them to know because they could help you deal with the illness?

If we keep our circle of the knowledgeable small, consider the likelihood that those we plan to tell will keep the information confidential. Recognize that telling someone significant information and then asking to keep it confidential places a burden on the person—a burden they may not want to bear. We have all heard things we wish we did not because we fear we will inadvertently release the information to others.

Few could argue against the position a spouse needs to know. Perhaps there might be some extenuating circumstances causing us to hold off bringing such news for a period, but a spouse has presumably observed the symptoms we have been struggling with and already knows something is wrong. Apart from exceptional circumstances, it is inconceivable we could journey well through life with a spouse we withheld such significant information from. On the other hand, there are important timing issues to consider when thinking about telling a romantic interest. If the long-term nature of one's relationship is in doubt, disclosing personal health information may not be appropriate—especially if we expect them to keep such information confidential if the relationship ends.

Children present a more complicated consideration. Factors such as their age, the illness's visibility, their ability to keep something confidential, and how the knowledge will impact them all must be assessed. While opinions differ, placing the burden of adult worries on children in their early years can create problems. Dealing with adult children who can't keep a confidence presents a special challenge that is difficult to navigate.

Whether to tell coworkers or our employer is a consideration to approach with special care. Telling coworkers while desiring to keep such information from our employer is fraught with risk. If requesting work accommodations, patients will need to confide in someone in the work environment. Before doing so, patients should educate themselves about employee rights under the Americans with Disabilities Act (available at www.ada.gov/). Many places of employment have a human resources (HR) department to assess and document the need for workplace accommodation. No one in a place of employment but HR needs to know about our specific ailment. The HR professional will determine the particular accommodations approved and inform our specific work unit of them. It is up to us whether to disclose anything further to our supervisor or coworkers. We have no obligation to satisfy the curiosity of fellow employees about what ails us.

A considerate (and legally compliant) supervisor will be careful not to put an employee in a position where they feel pressured to reveal the ailment to anyone apart from HR. The reality is not all supervisors function as they ought—so we need to think ahead of time how to respond if questions arise that make us feel we are being painted into a corner, and that revealing our ailment is the sole option for escape. However, if we have a sympathetic boss, we may find disclosure brings a level of understanding and flexibility that benefits our professional life.

One group must be told: health professionals who are caring for us. They are educated in and bound by law to keep health information confidential. Although we may think a particular issue is unassociated with the chronic ailment afflicting us, we will hinder a healthcare professional's ability to provide the optimum care if we withhold important health information. Sometimes we may need to deal with medical office staff not sensitive to the confidential nature of health information.

I had an appointment with an optometrist soon after I was diagnosed with MS. While I was standing at the office front desk, which was close to all the waiting patients, the receptionist asked me questions about my medical history. My responses would be heard by those nearby, so I told her I preferred to talk to the optometrist about those questions. When I met with him, I expressed my concern about the inability to discuss my medical history without others overhearing. He said he appreciated my bringing this concern to his attention and by the time of my next appointment, the outer office was restructured.

When to Tell

It is best for patients to come to grips with the reality and prognosis of the ailment before telling anyone outside of immediate family or a trusted counselor. We should learn about the ailment and prognosis before deciding whom to inform. Time will not always be on our side. But when time permits doing so, being slow and purposeful in these decisions is the best course of action.

Diagnostic uncertainty is one reason to not communicate a diagnosis to others. Awaiting the results of a second opinion or emergence of confirming symptoms will help us avoid the potential need to go back and correct previously communicated information. Greater certainty about our prognosis will enable us to better determine who and what to communicate.

What to Tell

Patients need to think carefully before telling someone, "I have an ailment, but I don't want to talk about it." There may be times when this is all we can or want to disclose, but realize we leave others to fill in the gaps with their imagination. We will likely face situations where we need to say something but desire to keep the content minimal.

Since there are studies showing a live attenuated vaccine like the one for yellow fever can exacerbate MS, I decided not to travel to countries where the yellow fever vaccine is recommended or required. A group of my faculty located in such a country repeatedly urged me to visit our site there, and it was reasonable to expect that, as dean of the college, I would do so. But I did not choose to reveal to any faculty I had been diagnosed with MS. Thus, my response to their urgings was simply, "I have a medical condition making it inadvisable for me to take the yellow fever vaccine. So, until this recommendation is lifted, I cannot visit." I struggled with whether I owed them a fuller explanation, but as health professionals, they understood the privacy of health information.

It is our decision as to how much information we want to disclose, and it is appropriate for us to expect others to respect the boundaries of information disclosure we have set. Realize we cannot hide information once it is disclosed, so be selective in what you say. Some patients find it helpful to create an elevator speech to summarize their condition on the fly. This is a concise statement of what the disease is and its expected alterations on our life. Having a summary in our head avoids the regret of walking away from an encounter wishing we had expressed things more clearly. It can also prevent us from sharing too much information.

In making a disclosure, we must recognize others will wonder how it should impact their interactions with us. If we will be open about the nature of our ailment, we should also be willing to address this inevitable question. Where appropriate, we should communicate how they can help. A trusted colleague can be an asset in helping us navigate the challenges of our ailment in the workplace.

A former colleague of mine had to undergo treatment with a biological medication known occasionally to induce personality changes. As was his right, he chose not to communicate to any of us his illness and the course of therapy he was undergoing. He developed substantial personality changes that detracted from his performance and made working with him difficult. He also struggled at home, where these changes were affecting his relationship with his wife. At some point, he revealed to a few of us his ailment and ongoing treatment. This enabled a forthright discussion of the personality changes we observed, of which he was unaware, and we could rally around him as colleagues to help him process this difficult period in his life. He benefited from disclosing his ailment and treatment to us.

This experience led me to choose to reveal my MS diagnosis to my personal assistant when I was starting treatment that could induce mood changes among other psychological adverse effects. Since so much of my day was spent at the university, any changes would likely show up there. I had a frank discussion with her, and my wife, about the potential psychological manifestations, requesting they watch for any behavioral changes. I was fortunate not to exhibit such adverse effects, but it was a comfort to me to have someone both at home and at work alert to the possibility and able to assist me if symptoms appeared.

How to Tell

There may be instances in which the decision to reveal our news arises spontaneously due to unforeseen circumstances. This is where having a concise summary in our heads can be especially useful. Preferably, however, we should think through just how we want to break the news and how much information to share. We cannot predict how people will respond to the news we share with them. Given this, we should avoid telling them in a setting where their reaction could draw undue attention and be hard to suppress. Sharing this news may also require more than one session. Especially for those who are close to us, time may be necessary to process the news before they can raise logical and appropriate questions.

It is appropriate to inform people who know about our condition that we desire to be the one to communicate this news to others. In the same vein, it is important to let those we do tell know who else knows. When the subject arises in the future, we may need to remind them of the parameters established—"Please remember you are the only one outside my immediate family who knows of my diagnosis. I would appreciate your continuing to keep this confidential."

We cannot predict how people will respond to such news, so it is best to avoid creating expectations for how they should respond. Like snowflakes, no two people are alike. People will respond differently to troubling news. Some will recoil and express how awful it is that we are facing this ailment. Others will hardly react to the news. Instead, they will take time to compute the impact of what you have told them. Patients should give each person the grace we would want to receive to respond in the context of their own personality and experiences. We need to be careful not to judge how much they care based on their initial response. Their caring will be demonstrated by their engagement with us over the long haul, not by their initial vocal or emotional response to the news we share.

Many, perhaps most, people will make an immediate association between the ailment and someone they have known with the same or similar disease. In truth, however, the single case they know of may not represent the usual experience for patients with this condition. As a consequence, some will have errant preconceived notions we may need to address. It is helpful to think ahead of time how to communicate the prognosis or likely impact of the illness.

As time progresses and we keep the circle of the knowing small, the probability that someone inadvertently discloses our illness increases. This may arise from one we have confided in. It is worth thinking ahead of time how to respond if this happens. I have a list in my head of those I would connect with if an accidental disclosure was likely to cause an uncontainable further release of this personal information. While I have had to deal with an unintended disclosure, I contained it quickly and continued to limit the circle of the knowing.

Regularly reevaluating the circle of those we inform is advisable for two reasons. First, both our ailment and relationships change over time. It is healthy to periodically assess whether there are others who should know, too. Second, it is a helpful reminder of who we have told. I did not create a master list of those I told initially, since the list was small, but I later wished I had. It may be helpful to create and maintain such a list so that we do not forget as time passes.

Words are impactful. This is why so many make a living as writers or public speakers. We have a certain measure of control over how the story of our ailment and its impact is communicated to the important people in our life. It is best to use this opportunity wisely.

CHAPTER 10

What to Do When New Symptoms Appear

Pain and weakness emerged on the area of my left forearm nearest the elbow. Writing for any length of time created an ache, making further efforts to hold a pen futile. The simple acts of lifting a coffee cup, opening a door, twisting a bottle cap, and tightening my shoelaces made me grimace and groan. I took the pain as a new symptom of MS, a sign of the ongoing deterioration of my nervous system. Since I expected further decline, I purchased a handbook intended for wounded warriors and began the process of learning to write like 90 percent of the population—right-handed. Trying to learn to write with my nondominant hand was frustrating and time consuming. I felt as though I had regressed to elementary school. Was this the beginning of progressive functional decline? Was I on the verge of losing my ability to do simple activities I had taken for granted for so long?

With the discomfort continuing to grow, my annual

appointment with my internist arrived. He listened carefully to my recent history of emerging symptoms. After pushing, pulling, and prodding my arm, he said, "I don't think this is a symptom of MS, I believe you have tendinitis." My response was one of surprise and pleasure. Perhaps this was one pain I would not need to live with for the rest of my days on this earth. Maybe it was not a harbinger of further decline.

Still, weeks of physical therapy provided no improvement. Referral to a local sports medicine specialist yielded a second opinion consistent with that of my internist—tendinitis. He stuck a needle into the most painful area and left a deposit of cortisone and local anesthetic. The injection eased the pain by a small degree for a short period. But my hope disappeared when the same symptoms developed and progressed with surprising speed in my right arm. This heightened the likelihood this might be an unusual symptom of MS. Soon, any use of my hands and arms sent jolts of pain streaking toward my torso. Shaking hands, something I did daily in my job, became almost unbearable.

My wife had recently had carpal tunnel surgery by a hand and elbow specialist. She suggested I get a second opinion from him. He cared for the elite athletes of professional sports teams and would-be athletes. Faced with continued deterioration, I was desperate to find relief. During the drive to Indianapolis for an appointment, my mind wandered back to the last time I visited a specialist who cared for professional athletes (recounted in chapter 1). That visit did not end well.

This specialist was everything one would desire in a surgeon. He was competent, compassionate, and conservative in his approach. Ultimately, this specialist performed the needed diagnostic assessment and identified the cause as tendinosis—a degeneration, rather than simple inflammation, of the deep tendon in both elbows. A year's worth of medical management failed to relieve my symptoms. This led to surgery in both arms to remove the 30 to 40 percent of each degenerated tendon. Before surgery, it was agony just to shave each day. Holding hands with my wife while walking created piercing pain. Postsurgery, I can do all those things and more with little discomfort. If I had continued assuming my symptoms arose from MS, my quality of life would be far less than it is today.

Responding to New Symptoms

Individuals with chronic ailments leading to physical deterioration face the challenge of discerning whether new symptoms represent another manifestation of their ongoing illness or an unrelated malady. It is not reasonable to run for an immediate clinical assessment with each new symptom. This is especially true when our provider is a specialist whose appointments are difficult to get or when the provider is far away.

How should those suffering from a chronic illness respond when new symptoms arise—or existing symptoms worsen? When is it time to get a skilled clinician to provide an evaluation? These are important questions to consider with care. Early in the course of a chronic illness, patients tend to seek an assessment for every new symptom that appears. As familiarity with the ailment and options for interventions gain ground, we are more inclined to ascribe new symptoms to progression and just bear it. Neither may be the best approach.

Any health professional will recommend patients with chronic illness see a clinician sooner rather than later. Even symptoms unrelated to our illness can exacerbate the underlying condition. We may also not respond as well to other illnesses due to our ongoing disease. This reality may lead to quicker treatment of other maladies to prevent potential exacerbations. At the same time, those of us living with chronic conditions also experience the normal symptoms of aging and mild maladies like everyone else. My current neurologist often reminds me, "MS patients get other ailments, just like people without MS." It is impractical for us to run for an evaluation with each new creak and groan in our bodies.

Since those living with an incurable chronic illness are often followed by a specialist (such as a neurologist or rheumatologist), it is advisable to have a candid discussion regarding what makes up an actionable change in our health. I must acknowledge that despite seeing many specialists over the years, none has ever brought this subject into the conversation. It has always required my prompting. Here is another place where we must be proactive.

The Discomfort of Ambiguity

While troubling for patients to realize, ambiguity in deciding whether emerging symptoms represent a relapse or progression of disease versus an unassociated phenomenon is a clinical reality. For example, researchers writing in the specialty journal *Multiple Sclerosis* reported substantial inconsistency among neurologists for exact criteria to determine whether a patient with MS is experiencing a relapse. Though disease-modifying drugs are used in MS patients to decrease the frequency of relapses, specialists are not uniform in their basis for labeling symptoms a relapse. If even specialists cannot agree, how is a patient to know? Unfortunately, patients with chronic illness cannot avoid this tension of uncertainty. We might wish it to be otherwise, but diagnostic ambiguity is unlikely to disappear soon. The complexity of our bodies and the effects of disease exceed human understanding.

Despite this ambiguity, patients need to learn how to decide when to seek further evaluation. Among things to consider are the following questions:

Is it a new symptom or an extension of ongoing symptoms?

Is the location in the body different from previous symptoms? Is the nature of the symptom different from what was experienced before (for example, previous symptoms were a dull ache; this is a lightning-like pulse of pain)? Is the timing or precipitating factor different (previous episodes occurred just at bedtime, but now they are happening midday)? Significant changes in the nature of the symptoms should prompt further evaluation from a clinician.

Is it persistent?

Pain, aches, soreness, tingling sensations, and numbness occasionally occur in otherwise healthy individuals. They often last hours, even a day or two, and then disappear. Our bodies are both wonderful and weird. We would be under constant medical evaluation if we sought help for every odd feeling that pops up in our bodies. Obviously, a large difference exists between a sudden inability to walk and a new slight itch in your nose. We all recognize the former as a medical emergency, while the latter is best ignored. But what about symptoms that fall between these two extremes?

Most strange feelings resolve without intervention. A key to deciding whether something needs an evaluation is persistence. Nevertheless, how long does one observe symptoms before seeking help? No simple answer exists for this question, as the nature of the symptoms are important. Usually, a day or two of observation is advisable. Over this brief course of time, are the symptoms stable or progressing? Symptoms that become more intense, increase in a certain area, or impair normal activity deserve a skilled evaluation. Stable or slowly resolving symptoms need more time for observation.

Is it expected within the spectrum of what is known about the ailment?

Variation in the intensity and nature of symptoms is an expected part of the normal course of some diseases. For example, patients with MS often find sensory symptoms intensify as their body temperature rises. Increased symptoms in hot weather or with exercising are expected and do not require a medical evaluation. Patients with trigeminal neuralgia experience increased pain in times of stress. This increase in pain does not indicate disease progression or therapy failure but is part of the impact on the day-to-day life for such patients. The need to recognize these normal variations in disease symptoms is an important reason patients should educate themselves about their disease. It helps them differentiate the expected from the unexpected. It may also help them determine when to see a specialist versus a primary care provider.

A specialist is best equipped to evaluate new symptoms or a significant extension of existing symptoms normally associated with a chronic ailment. A primary care provider is better suited to provide the first evaluation of symptoms not consistent with the underlying disease. Our primary care provider may also be knowledgeable about our chronic illness. If they have seen a significant number of patients with the ailment over time, they may be comfortable assessing disease flare-ups. This is a topic to discuss with our primary care provider as we think through how to manage our chronic illness over the long haul.

Accessibility may also determine whether we consult a specialist or primary care provider. The latter is most likely local, while the former is sometimes distant. The ease of access may make our primary care provider the first stop for evaluating all new symptoms, regardless of the likelihood they are manifestations of our chronic ailment.

Is there an intervention that may reduce its impact?

One consideration in responding to new or worsening symptoms is the availability of options for medical interventions. For example, relapses or flare-ups of many autoimmune and inflammatory diseases respond to a course of corticosteroids (such as prednisone). While these potent drugs can be effective for such flare-ups, they produce significant adverse effects—both short- and long-term. Some patients will forgo treatment for mild flare-ups rather than bear these adverse effects. These choices require educated consideration, including consultation with the appropriate specialist—as the cumulative effect of multiple flares of a degenerative disease may significantly impact long-term functioning.

Disease-modifying drugs slow the decline or frequency of flare-ups in some diseases, such as rheumatoid arthritis, MS, lupus, and certain inflammatory bowel diseases. A patient who experiences multiple flares while on one agent may be advised to switch to a different agent to reduce the frequency of worsening symptoms. Thus, for some patients, it is important to alert a specialist so they can assess the severity and frequency of flares as it may cause a change in ongoing therapy.

Is it changing things important in our life?

An annoyance should be responded to differently than a functional deficit that impairs our normal activity. The intensity of pain, numbness, fatigue, or lightheadedness is not as important as its impact on our life. If the new or worsened symptom causes a meaningful change in activities we perform regularly, it merits a clinician's assessment.

Patients may view some symptoms as an annoyance that, in fact, may have long-term implications if not addressed. It does not take long before a sudden sleep impairment causes sleep deprivation, leading to a decline in our overall well-being. Symptoms impairing sexual activity can affect the relationship most important to us. Difficulty swallowing may seem like an annoyance, but if it provokes a change in our diet, it can have extended effects on our health. Dizziness may seem to be nothing more than a bother, but if it results in a fall, the implications can be far reaching. The point is this: we should not dismiss new symptoms too quickly. We need to think about the implications of leaving them unaddressed. This will help us assess the need for intervention. When in doubt, get it checked out.

Some patients are hesitant to contact their specialist because they don't want to bother a busy clinician. This should never be a reason for not seeing a specialist who is helping to manage our care. First, recognize most clinicians have time built into their schedules for patients with acute needs. We are not a disruption to their schedule. They have staff devoted to managing their schedule to deal with needs like ours. Admittedly, some office staff are more helpful in times of need than others. Occasionally, we may need to be a forceful advocate for ourselves to get past personnel barriers. If such barriers do arise, it is important to communicate these problems to our specialist. They do not know how the office staff is responding unless we share our experience with them.

Second, don't assume your perception reflects that of your clinician. Just because you are concerned they will consider your visit a bother does not mean they will. Their professional career is devoted to caring for patients like us. Many have selected their specialty because they find professional satisfaction dealing with complex cases. Our need may end up being the most interesting part of their day.

Finally, if they do respond to your visit with actions that are less than caring, think carefully about why this happened. Is it out of character for them? We all have bad days, which we sometimes project onto those we interact with. If their response is unusual, cut them the same slack you would want in their shoes. However, if it is a pattern in their interactions with you, it may be time to consider a new specialist. You need the help of a clinician who will work with you to manage your disease. If they do not welcome your visit to seek their expert advice, you need to find a partner who will.

How are we responding emotionally to the new or worsening symptom?

We should not underestimate the emotional impact of uncertainty when new symptoms arise or progressive symptoms worsen. If we fixate on the new development—brooding about what it portends—it is important to get a skilled clinical assessment. Rather than allowing our minds to cogitate on the what-ifs, it is best to get a settled opinion about what is going on within our bodies. Worry is both draining and unproductive. It can distract us from things we should be giving attention to. When it arises over new symptoms, this should be reason enough to seek medical advice.

In contrast, some patients are inclined to passive avoidance. They'd rather not know things are getting worse and the disease is progressing. But we're fooling ourselves if we think not knowing is better. Avoiding the truth will not halt progression. We have all heard of people who ignored important symptoms and did not seek help until it was too late to do anything. Following in their footsteps is not a path to living well.

One challenge of homeownership is learning when a thump, squeak, crack, or drip means it is time to call a repair specialist. Misjudgments in this area can cause bigger and more costly problems. The same is true with our physical selves. A thoughtful approach to dealing with new or extended symptoms is essential to thriving in the face of a chronic ailment.

CHAPTER 11

Dealing with the Regret of Choices That Harm Your Health

The only sounds breaking the silence of the moments past midnight were the beeps coming from the monitor above my daughter's bed. They confirmed her heart rate and rhythm, blood pressure, and respirations were fine. Despite these positive signs, she appeared as one wrung out like a wet washcloth. My beautiful girl had undergone six hours of abdominal surgery. A general surgeon made an incision from her navel to almost the middle of her back. He then lifted out her kidney and other organs to enable the spinal surgeon to insert a rod and screws in the front of her spine. Seeing her in the recovery room afterward pierced my heart with anguish.

As I stood beside her bed gently caressing her cheek hours later, the charge entering my consciousness brought tears to my eyes. This same charge surfaced in the weeks leading up to this moment. Only now, standing in the aftermath of the surgeons' intricate work to straighten her spine, the guilt struck me more powerfully than ever. "This is your fault," the accusing inner voice charged. "You could have prevented this. You're her father. You were supposed to watch over and protect her, but you failed miserably here."

My daughter needed a physical to play soccer in high school. Her regular pediatrician was on maternity leave, and the one filling in for her did the simple exam I assumed was done each year during her physical. As my daughter bent over and the pediatrician examined her spine, she told my wife it appeared our daughter had scoliosis. The degree of the curvature did not appear too severe, but she referred us to a specialist nonetheless.

Childhood memories surfaced in my mind in the weeks leading to the appointment. A young girl my age underwent spinal surgery to correct scoliosis. She spent months restrained in a body cast. I recalled images of her parents wheeling her to our community pool strapped on a board with four wheels. She would lie on this board for hours while her brothers swam. Thinking of my daughter in such a state for months on end made me shudder. I devoted countless hours to scouring the medical literature for the latest recommendations for managing scoliosis, in particular the criteria for surgery. My wife and I carefully assessed the specialist we were referred to—including getting the opinions of orthopedic surgeons we knew who focused on other parts of the body. We asked a common question: "If it were your daughter, who would you want to do the surgery?"

We arrived at the appointed day and time to meet with the Harvard-trained spinal specialist. A sense of relief came when his physical exam suggested the curvature was minor. He cautioned us that some patients mask an extensive curve well and an X-ray was necessary to be sure. To the annoyance of my wife and daughter, I paced nonstop as we waited for the specialist to return after the X-rays. Unfortunately, my daughter masked the misshaped spine well. The curvature was severe, and she needed surgery.

I struggled emotionally with this verdict more than any of my own diagnoses, especially since the surgery would have been unnecessary if the curve was caught early. She would have slept in a restrictive brace designed to prevent the curve from increasing. Why did I not ask if her spine had been checked during the many appointments her regular pediatrician examined her? I battled a haunting voice within me in the weeks leading up to her surgery. The hours I spent at her bedside and months of recovery with limited mobility brought anguishing battles with self-blame. As she has experienced pain over the years from the implanted rod, at times debilitating, I struggled with deep regret of what might have been if I had been proactive, making sure her spine was checked annually. No objective arguments or rational explanations will ever fully free me of the regret and sense I could have spared her what will probably be a lifetime of discomfort.

The Agony of Regret

Living with the question of "what if only I had or had not?" is common. A career decision gone sour. A romantic interest turned ugly. Money lost in an ill-advised investment. A move to a new town that did not meet expectations. For some, a careless, unwise, or foolish action has led to a life with an unremitting ailment.

Patients who acquired AIDS through sexual contact may be haunted by the immeasurable impact of their sexual choices. Some patients with emphysema are plagued with the knowledge that their choice to smoke caused their ailment. Others who live with lost eyesight from diabetes beat themselves up over their neglect to manage their disease carefully. Patients disabled from an accident find their mind drawn to questions about choices they made leading up to the accident, while those with injuries arising from medical interventions will spend years kicking themselves for agreeing to undergo the procedure.

For example, Julie lived with unrelenting, intense pain from a benign tumor on her spine. Specialists recommended a procedure likely to sever her spinal cord. While it would leave her a paraplegic, they were confident it would end the pain torturing her for the last decade. Desperate to find relief, she agreed to the surgery. As expected, the resulting surgery left her paralyzed from the waist down. But it did not reduce her pain at all. Consequently, she faced the rest of her life not only in chronic pain, but also with the limitations and complications paralysis brought to her body. Her suffering was increased by the deep regret of having agreed to the surgical intervention.

The impact on and frequency of regret among patients is poorly understood. Yet, as Drs. Jerome Groopman and Pamela Hartzband noted in a perceptive piece in the *New England Journal of Medicine*, "self-blame can be one of the greatest burdens in a patient's life." It is hard to live with the knowledge you (or someone else) could have prevented the suffering you now endure. Investigators have found that patients who blame themselves for an injury-producing accident do not cope as well with their physical challenges as others who do not blame themselves.

For others, their choice or lack thereof has altered the course of someone else's health. Perhaps the most profound examples come from health professionals whose errors caused serious physical harm to patients. Physicians involved in serious errors report increased stress and sleeping difficulties. Health professionals whose actions inadvertently harm patients may develop symptoms consistent with posttraumatic stress disorder (PTSD). The depth of agony for some is so great they leave their profession—and a few even commit suicide. Such is the intensity of their personal torture from regretting choices they made.

Regret can be a powerful emotion. Left unaddressed, it chews at our insides like termites in wood. This is particularly true when the consequences of our regretful action continue—consequences like a chronic ailment or disability. The persistent physical reminder of one's choice can act like a dripping faucet, sending a repeated ping to your mind and preventing you from putting aside the ill-conceived action. We cannot undo the past, but we must come to grips with it. It is the only way to live well.

Responding to Feelings of Regret

There are some key steps to living well in the face of regretful choices that impact our health:

Avoid Misplaced Blame. First, we should *determine if our regret is legitimate*. In other words, is there anything we could have done to prevent our ailment? Some patients embrace self-blame when no evidence is available that their actions caused their ill health. A host of self-help health gurus on the scene today argue all or most disease is caused by errant thinking or coping with life. One well-known health advocate has argued you can control 95 percent of the genetic mutations leading to cancer and autoimmune diseases through right living. Buying into this philosophy, some patients even blame their cancer on their own negative emotions and expressions. While much about the mind-body interface remains a mystery—and emotions can provoke or worsen physical symptoms—definitive evidence that disease is caused by, or prevented through, our thinking and emotions is lacking.

Misplaced self-blame results in self-harm. It can create a life-draining despondency and impair our ability to cope well with illness. Those with intense feelings of self-blame will often generalize: "My blame in this instance shows I am a worthless person. I always make wrong and harmful choices." Researchers reported findings in the *Journal of Affective Disorders* that indicate self-blame is significantly associated with major depressive disorder. Those caught in a destructive pattern of self-blame should seek professional or spiritual counsel.

When a thoughtful assessment leads to the conclusion that regret is not legitimate, such regret should be dismissed. Continued questioning over our role in the adverse outcome is unhealthy and should not be entertained. Just like it is unwise for us to travel to certain places physically, it is also advisable to avoid traveling certain paths mentally. Repeatedly reassessing our role in a chronic condition's development is one such path to avoid.

Focus on What You Can Change. If you conclude you bear some measure of responsibility, determine if *you can make it right.* The answer is most likely no. Decisions leading to adverse health effects can rarely be undone. But is there anything we can do now that will make a difference? Perhaps we developed adult onset diabetes because of poor dietary choices over the years. Embracing a sound diet and regular exercise can bring a measure of blood glucose control and reduce the need for medications, as well as minimize the disease's consequences. While the choice to smoke may have led to emphysema, quitting now can make a difference in our current and future breathing ability—as well as reduce the risk of stroke or heart attack. We should focus on what we can do rather than on unchangeable past choices.

Seek to Learn from the Experience. If we cannot make a difference in terms of the specific health issue, what lesson can we learn to apply to future life choices? The decision or action contributing to our illness is just one of many decisions we would make differently based on what we know today. In truth, we all make unwise choices with lasting impact. Most of us do so repeatedly. Some declined a career opportunity which hindsight reveals would have led to tremendous professional success and satisfaction. Others have unwisely purchased a home without performing due diligence and are left with cash- and time-draining repairs. Still others have made choices damaging a valued relationship. Life often presents us with opportunities to learn from our failures.

This is part of life. Responding to our failures is more important in molding us as people than our successes. Anyone who honestly reflects on their life will find many instances of choices they would handle differently today. Our frailty as humans includes our imperfection in decision-making. Sometimes this imperfection impacts our health.

Some whose choices led to serious health consequences use their experience as a platform to educate others. Smokers whose habit resulted in emphysema or cancer have sought to warn young people of the dangers of smoking. Former NBA star Magic Johnson chose to use his HIV positive diagnosis and celebrity status to assist in public education about AIDS. I recently listened to a teen who used her horrendous car accident as a platform to warn peers of the dangers of texting while driving. Working to spare others the same experience of regret may benefit some patients.

Refuse to Dwell on It. We cannot rescind past choices. We should learn from the past but resist the temptation to dwell on it. Not brooding over past decisions is a choice of the will. We must consciously refuse to allow our mind to focus on the matter. When such thoughts enter your head unprompted, dismiss them as an unwanted guest and actively focus your attention elsewhere. This is hard to accomplish. Dark and depressing thinking seems to grip us more readily than things that are beautiful, encouraging, and healthy. But just as we can train and strengthen a muscle, we can actively train our minds toward healthy responses to unprovoked thoughts of regret.

I have often used a simple exercise with people. I ask them not to think about pink elephants. Whatever you do, I tell them, I don't want you to think about pink elephants. Simply do not allow the thought of pink elephants to enter your mind. Of course, whenever I do this, people can't help but think of pink elephants. The point is that you will not rid yourself of thoughts by telling yourself not to think about them. Such an exercise simply solidifies the matter in your mind. This is known as an ironic process—trying to suppress thoughts about something makes you more likely to think about it. Instead, you must turn your mind elsewhere. You must learn to redirect your thoughts when things arise that you wish to avoid dwelling on. This means developing a plan as to how and to what you will turn your thinking.

Avoid Dwelling on the Blame of Others. It should also be noted that blaming others creates a destructive cycle. While some seem to think finding someone to blame is salutary, studies actually find individuals who blame others for their severe injury cope more poorly with the consequences of their illness. Thus, while others may be at fault, brooding on the blame is counterproductive to our well-being. Dwelling on what could have been is not only painful, it also paralyzes our ability to make the most of the present and future.

Anyone who has received forgiveness from another knows how freeing this gift feels. To be forgiven a wrongdoing that you have acknowledged is an incomparable experience. Some of the most precious and closest moments in my relationship with my wife have come when she has forgiven me for thoughtless and hurtful things I have said. Her gift of forgiveness has not only freed me from feelings of guilt, it has also revealed the depth of her love for me.

It is also a powerful freeing experience to grant

forgiveness to another. Granting forgiveness can prevent a root of bitterness from strangling our soul. If our illness or injury is caused by the actions or inaction of another, it is in our best interest to grant forgiveness and move on. Above all, avoiding brooding in anger over the harm is the path to living well.

Akeyo is a woman who exemplifies this reality. I met her some years ago on the outskirts of a town in sub-Saharan Africa on her small passion fruit farm. Her beaming smile and exuberant movements as she showed off her growing harvest gave no hint of the painful reality she lived with. She was infected with HIV by a promiscuous husband who left the scene long ago. Without the program President Bush initiated to provide medications for HIV-infected people in sub-Saharan Africa, her diagnosis would have been a certain death sentence. Medication keeps her alive, but it provides no cure. She lives with the perpetual risk of the virus developing resistance to the medications. With a perspective rooted in her faith, she gave no place to bitterness at her lot in life. In contrast is Ricardo, who lost a son in a tragic automobile accident because of another driver's careless actions. Bitterness consumed his life and drove away fellow members of his small-town community. His response left him a lonely, isolated person. He went to his grave embittered by his loss.

The lesson is simple. Harm may have come our way through the actions of another, but how we respond will determine the depth of that harm.

Putting Regret in Perspective

Life is an endless series of choices. Some are rather inconsequential, while others can be life changing. Even when they are made with substantial care, hindsight often reveals we don't make the best choices. This is part of our fallibility as humans. What is important is learning to productively deal with the regret of choices. The past is unchangeable. The future is unpredictable. But it is within our power to determine how we respond to the tension both produce in the present. This is how we land on the path to thriving instead of the road leading to remorse.

CHAPTER 12

How Can Those Who Care Help?

A package arrived at my house unexpected and unwanted. It was a small box wrapped in brown paper and delivered by our faithful mailwoman. The surface and shape of the innocuous brown box gave no hints of its contents. With no recent or upcoming birthday or anniversary, I could not imagine what the sender enclosed. My heart sank as I opened the package and extracted the contents. The sender's intention was good—more than good, actually. It arose out of an earnest desire to help from someone who loved me. In reality, the gesture was not helpful. Contained within this box was yet another misguided attempt from a well-meaning person to provide me what they were certain was a cure for my ailments. The product lacked any scientific evidence of health benefit, and its production quality was unknown. The sender expected I would take this substance while in a fragile health state with a perturbed immune system, with their assurance this product would help me turn the corner health-wise.

I would be a rich man if I had gained a dollar every time someone approached me with what they were sure was a remedy for what ailed me. Like others, I learned to dread encounters with such persons. How do you politely decline their uninformed medical advice? Experiences like this make those who suffer from chronic ailments hesitate to inform others of their health struggles. Like Job's friends—who prompted him to declare "miserable comforters are you all"— others often add to the suffering rather than provide relief or encouragement in the struggle.

Those who live with chronic ailments learn all too quickly that most people are unsure how to help others who are suffering. Sometimes the efforts to help are clumsy, and other times they bring further discomfort. Human foolishness being what it is, such encounters are inevitable for those who suffer. Learning to deal with them is imperative for one's sanity.

Those who suffer from chronic ailments must learn how to address heartfelt and well-meaning questions that hold different implications in the context of our experience. What should I say when someone asks me, "How are you?" If I were transparent, on a *normal* day, I would need to say, "Well, half my face feels like it is being pricked by a thousand needles, the bottom of both feet burn like they are on fire, my lower left leg seems to be encased in ever-shrinking cement, my back aches, and I'm exhausted because I only got two to three hours of sleep each night for the last several weeks." I concluded long ago such transparency is not a good idea—though I have been tempted a time or two to test the reaction of the questioner to such an honest response. Obviously, it would be unkind to do a verbal body slam on someone who is well-meaning but unaware of the full context and implications of their question. Rather, I find such moments to be a good reminder to show more thought in my choice of words to others. I retain enough stupidity in me to need such reminders, and there seems to be no shortage of others willing to provide it.

If you wish to help someone suffering a chronic ailment, what should you say to them? What should you not say? What can you do to be helpful? What should you avoid? Let's start with what not to say or do.

Don't Pretend You Know How They Feel

The suffering provoked by chronic ailments is not like an Egg McMuffin from McDonald's—with identical appearance, taste, and texture no matter the location. The same ailment affects people differently and changes over time. Suffering arises from the interplay of physical, emotional, and spiritual inputs. You cannot know how another person feels unless they communicate their experience to you. Often, one suffering cannot even articulate their experience amid their suffering. So, if you want to be a helper, do not let the words "I know how you feel" escape from your lips. Banish this phrase to the land of "say no more." You may intend to make the person aware that you empathize with their experience, but the words will sound dismissive and arrogant. At best, they will be unhelpful.

Don't Play the Comparison Game

As my back injury profoundly reduced my ability to sit, my struggle with back pain was clear to those I lived life with, both personally and professionally. The same scene played out so many times it became predictable. I'd be standing in a meeting or other gathering when everyone else was sitting. Before, during, or after the event, someone nearby would turn and say, "Bad back, eh?" After I would affirm their Sherlock Holmes–like deduction, they would respond with something such as, "Yeah, I get a tweak in my back every now and then too."

Really? A tweak every now and then? My back hurt so bad I was on the verge of tears. I had not taken a vacation with my family in years because I could not tolerate the sitting required to travel. I couldn't even enjoy a dinner out with my wife because I was unable to sit through dinner in a restaurant. Having someone tell me they also get a tweak in their back now and then didn't suggest they sympathized with my plight—which they clearly didn't comprehend. What is worse is that I, who have been on the receiving end of such comparisons, have made similar pointless and insensitive comments of comparison myself. For several years I have watched people with an obvious physical ailment (such as an injured arm in a sling) interact and concluded that trying to compare someone's health issue with one of our own is a popular past-time.

Playing the comparison game is unhelpful. In fact, it is self-centered. Instead of expressing empathy to the sufferer, it draws attention to ourselves. Do you want to help chronic sufferers? Commit yourself to avoiding making comparisons between their ailment and your personal experience.

Don't Give Unsolicited Medical Advice

I could fill a book with the amount of unsolicited medical advice I have received over the years, much of it unsound and equal portions of it misguided. It is amazing how quick people who know so little about you are to give medical advice. Many patients keep their ailment hidden to avoid the barrage of unsolicited advice sure to follow disclosure. I'd make a simple plea to those who want to be helpful: do not give unsolicited medical advice. Just don't do it.

An individual with an incurable chronic ailment has most likely intensively scoured the earth for a solution to their physical dilemma. They have seen experts, read all they could, and spoken to others with the same ailment or a similar one. Those who know them best have often also taken part in the desperate search for a solution. For someone else to arrive on the scene with scant information and a lack of medical expertise to pronounce the route to a cure is, well, rather brash and foolish. Best to keep your thoughts to yourself.

Don't Tell People You Hope They Feel Better Soon

It is difficult for people with chronic illness to respond to good wishes when they know they will *never* get better. In fact, barring some unforeseen medical advance or miracle, as time progresses, the sufferers will only feel worse. A chronic ailment is not like the common cold wherein improvement is inevitable. Therefore, our response to people with these two issues should not be the same.

Don't Assume What They Can or Cannot Do

If you want an eye-opening exercise, next time you experience a delayed flight in an airport, spend some time sitting in a wheelchair and see how people interact with you. People will speak louder, thinking your presumed inability to walk must also have impaired your hearing. Others will speak to you as if you have mentally regressed to childhood. Everything about your appearance screams you are an adult, but others engage you as if whatever caused you to need a wheelchair has also taken away your cognitive ability. It is remarkable how being identified as having an ailment causes people to assume all kinds of things about us. Avoid making such assumptions. Where relevant, simply ask. Most people will appreciate your thoughtfulness.

Don't Expect Them to Always Avoid Increasing Their Own Discomfort

Like many chronic sufferers, I don't remember what it is like to wake up without pain. I have learned to live with pain as a constant companion and recognize the things that will cause this unwanted guest to make more noise than usual. While there are times its noise-making is too disturbing to bear, other times I will accept its increased volume as a part of the journey. I will deliberately and willingly do things I expect to make the pain worse. To do otherwise would be to limit my quality of life unacceptably. I cannot live avoiding everything that increases my pain.

Loved ones often find this hard to accept, and their compassion for those with illness would prefer they avoid anything provoking increased discomfort. But those who care must allow sufferers to select the boundaries of their activity and accept their choices of activities they know will temporarily increase their suffering. There are times those closest to the person in pain should initiate a frank discussion about the wisdom of particular activity choices. In general, those who wish to help need to give space to let those with chronic ailments make what are truly painful choices.

Now that I have provided a series of things not to do or say, you might conclude that it would be safer to avoid those with chronic ailments rather than risk offending them through inappropriate words or actions. It would be a disservice if my advice drew you to such a decision. Isolation is one of the worst consequences for chronic sufferers.

Life is messy, because people's lives are messy. Your neighbor, Cassie, may not suffer from a chronic ailment, but she battles the scars of childhood abuse. Your coworker, Juan, may not live with constant physical pain, but he is living with the heart-wrenching agony of a failing marriage. Your boss, Emma, does not have an increasing physical disability, but her life is consumed with caring for a mother who no longer recognizes her. Rare is the individual who is not facing some significant challenge in their life. And if they are spared such challenges for the time being, a train wreck they don't even know about is likely coming around the corner. Those suffering with chronic illnesses are not different from others you engage with; they are fellow humans on this journey we call life making their unique contributions and having their own special challenges. The human experience is enriched when we take the time and effort to journey together well.

So, how can we engage with chronic sufferers in a way that helps, or at least does not add to their burden?

Compassion

One of the more humorous television commercials of recent years featured an NFL star quarterback at the counter of a coffee shop. When the barista collapses on the floor after inadvertently scalding himself with steam, the NFL star leans over, urges him to "rub some dirt on it," and encourages him to move on. It is humorous precisely because it is the wrong thing to say at the moment. The lack of compassion is self-evident.

All who suffer with a chronic ailment frequently need to give themselves a pep talk to not allow their ailment to limit their activity unnecessarily, and such words may rightly be spoken by those who know them best. However, compassion is the best response from most people they encounter. Not pity, but compassion. People who suffer chronically don't want our pity or even sympathy, but they do need our understanding.

True compassion arises out of sincere concern for others. It arises from a heart able to put others before themselves. The heart attitude is the most important element for displays or responses of compassion. Rather than becoming overly analytical about what we should say or do for a friend who is a chronic sufferer, developing a heart of concern for others will enable the practical outworking of compassion to flow with ease.

We live in a culture that urges the car in front of us to get out of our way so we can get where we are going more quickly. Impatience grows within us on a plane as we await the people from the seats in front of us to deboard so we can get on our way. We fidget with impatience in the grocery store checkout line when the person in front of us with many items causes us to wait longer before we are checked out and on our way. People we encounter are more often seen as obstacles to our objective rather than fellow citizens to whom we are inextricably tied.

The afternoon my wife and I made arrangements at the funeral home after the tragic death of our youngest son, we stopped at the grocery store to pick up some essential items we could not put off. The experience was surreal. We were two deeply wounded people who felt so out of place and disconnected from our surroundings. Both of us were on the verge of tears as we conducted our necessary business. As we waited for our turn at the cashier, I wondered how often I'd unknowingly been in line behind someone in the midst of a similarly traumatic experience or even one in intense physical pain. Had I always been so self-consumed that I gave no thought to anything but my pace of moving through the line?

We live in an era where self-centeredness is treated as a virtue. The endless self-aggrandizement by many athletes, celebrities, and politicians feeds this warped view of humanity. Advertizers appeal to our self-interests to convince us happiness is unattainable apart from their product. The selfie generation struggles to be the focal point of every picture. Such a focus is incongruent with compassion for our fellow humans.

Compassion is a virtue that does not come naturally. It requires us to battle against our own self-interests and develop a mindset that truly cares about the suffering of those around us. This is why those who have suffered a serious loss themselves tend to be more compassionate than those who have been spared such pain. In my life, nothing has made me more conscious of and sensitive to the suffering of others than my personal experiences of suffering. It is hard to comprehend the depth and breadth of suffering if you have been spared such experiences in your own life.

At a social engagement many years ago, guests at the table were asked to share what they did professionally. After I described my professional activity as a biomedical researcher, another guest with the sniffles recommended I shift my energy to finding a cure for the common cold. While the comment provoked chuckles from the other guests, I replied by saying I hope we never find a cure for the common cold. One who incredulously asked, "Why would you hope for that?" broke the stunned silence of the dinner guests. I replied that the common cold is the only ailment most young health professionals have personally experienced. Unlike all generations before the second half of the twentieth century, they likely never even experienced an immediate family member dying from an infectious disease. How much empathy would they have for those suffering from illness if we took away the common cold?

If you want to help those who suffer from chronic illness, develop a compassionate heart for those around you. Consider the impact of your own experiences of suffering. Regularly undertake the exercise of thinking beyond yourself and enter into the experiences of others. This may take the form of empathetically questioning those who suffer so you can better understand their life experience. It may mean becoming a more careful observer of those around you.

How do we become more empathetic? We are unlikely to do so by a simple determination of the will. But there are ways to open our eyes and hearts to the experience of others. Here is where the power of story can help us. Many who have experienced the suffering brought by chronic illness have taken up the pen and opened a window into their lives. Their recorded experiences help us better understand the life journey of others.

Sometimes the best compassion comes from devoting the time to listen with care. We have all experienced moments of relief just by getting something off our chest. Simply declaring our struggle seems to remove swelling tension. When a friend or colleague shares such struggles, we have a strong inclination to suggest a path to fix the problem. Rarely, if ever, does this truly meet a need. We humans seem to need to know there are others who recognize our struggle. Rather than wanting us to fix their problem, those suffering often want a listening ear from someone who cares. They seek nothing more from us. And we gain greater understanding by listening to them.

Chronic Courtesy

A courtesy is a respectful or considerate act. Call it an act of kindness if you prefer. A considerate person will hold the door open for someone whose arms are filled. They will pick up an unnoticed dropped item and return it to its rightful owner. They will assist someone who has tripped and spilled the contents of their shopping bag. Able-bodied individuals have momentary needs where such courtesies are deeply appreciated. Those suffering from chronic illnesses will often need chronic courtesy. These small acts of kindness are one way you can provide meaningful help to chronic sufferers.

One dear friend who joins us for regular gatherings in our home returns chairs to their normal location in our living room at the end of each gathering. He knows lifting heavy chairs is unwise for me and kindly takes on this task so I can avoid stressing my body. It is a small but very helpful gesture. It takes him a minute or two, but it saves me increased pain each night of our gathering. I didn't ask him to do this. In fact, I would never have asked him to do so. But he regularly engages in courtesies like this because he has developed a compassionate heart and seems to always be on the lookout for opportunities to meet the needs of others. In fact, his pattern of helping without asking has made me more willing to ask for help. It has also made me more observant of opportunities to help others myself.

If you know one who suffers chronically, be alert to ways you can make their journey just a little bit easier. When we observe an opportunity, it may be wise to ask, "Would it help if I . . .?" Some things may appear helpful on the surface but in reality are less than helpful.

But won't this put demands on our time and energy? Yes, it will. Nevertheless, I am confident we will find it far more rewarding personally than many other ways we could spend our time. If all of us devoted small amounts of time doing small acts of courtesy for those in need, our society would be a far different place to live in. Actually, it would probably be a better place to live in.

For those who suffer from chronic ailments, it is important to realize that our journey of pain or other limitation does not place us in the special position of always being the recipient of courtesy. We have the means and opportunity to do likewise for others, and we should do so. In addition, it is important to think about how we respond to those who offer their help. Wanting to be independent and not seen as needy, we can respond in a discourteous manner (*The nerve of them thinking I need their help!*). Not only is this rude to the individual, but this reaction probably discourages them from offering help to others. Be humble enough to accept the kind courtesies of others.

Connectedness

As I have journeyed through the series of ailments described in this book, it is hard to imagine what the experience would be like without my soulmate, my dear wife of over three and a half decades. She had little idea of the full implications when she promised to be with me in sickness and in health. She has seen in me more of the former than the latter. Her companionship, encouragement, patience, and simple presence have been of immeasurable help. Family, friends, and colleagues have also been important to my living well in the face of chronic suffering.

People with chronic ailments need to feel connected to others. They need to know their ailment has not broken the bonds of friendship and other relationships that make life so worth living. They need to be involved and engaged in the lives of others. Recently, considerable attention has been drawn to the negative health implications of loneliness, which may be as impactful as tobacco smoking. Some have even called the level of loneliness in our society an epidemic.

Yet increasing physical limitations experienced by those with chronic illnesses often present special challenges to remaining socially connected. If we know of another's limitations, we should keep them in mind as we plan activities that would include them. For example, in choosing a restaurant to meet a group at, do we consider whether it is accessible for our friend in a wheelchair? If they feel progressive fatigue as the day wears on, do we try to plan such outings early enough to encourage their engagement? It is easy for those experiencing escalating physical disability to pull away from social engagements that are increasingly difficult. Anything we can do to reduce the barriers will help them stay connected.

Many in our society face increasing limitations in their physical abilities and have no one they can count on being there as their ailment progresses. They live alone. There may be no family to watch over them. They represent a very special needs group in our society that is growing in number. A program or a system of care will not meet their needs. It is in the context of

else on the field was indiscernible to him.

Similarly, the lens through which you see the world has a remarkable influence on how you respond to the inevitable tribulations of life. This lens influences what you see and how you see it. It also determines how you interpret what is happening to you both from within and from without. The lens through which I see the world has not only shaped my response to the challenges I have shared within these pages, but it has also shaped this book itself. This gets to the heart of the matter.

Any author must define their audience and, through the innumerable revisions of their manuscript, assure their text keeps its focus on those expected readers. As I embarked on the literary journey of producing this book, I had to decide whether I would direct my words to all those whose journey in life included an uninvited pathological companion, or focus on those who also shared a spiritual path similar to the one I have charted in my life. I focused on the former out a desire to help as many as possible. I am grateful to live in a pluralistic society where all citizens are free to chart their own faith journey—and one in which the marketplace of ideas is open to all to put forth their views. At the same time, the story of my journey is incomplete without acknowledging the spiritual element serving as the compass throughout most of my earthly passage— most particular in my decades of physical affliction. As I believe thriving in the face of suffering is primarily a matter of the heart, it would be less than honest not to share this element of my life. It forms the basis of my hope in the face of affliction.

When an individual faces the hard reality that their illness or suffering will endure, the focus often moves from the body to their personhood. We view an acute illness as a problem with our physical selves. The pain, shortness of breath, dizziness, or other symptoms will pass once healing takes place. The body will recover and the suffering will cease. But when suffering becomes permanent, our personhood is greatly impacted—often becoming the most intense locus of suffering. Physical limitations bring about changes in our role in life. How we perceive ourselves, and are viewed by others, can alter dramatically. These changes are often more painful than the physical elements of our illness. The loss brings sorrow and, sometimes, a crisis of identity.

To navigate the troubled waters these changes bring, we need a compass for our heart. Without one, like a ship that has lost the north star, we bounce around in the storms our illness brings. Before illness struck, we viewed ourselves as self-sufficient—needing no navigator to assist us in life. Chronic suffering teaches us otherwise. Likely, we will find ourselves searching for a safe harbor and source of hope.

Hope is the seed from which victorious living can grow in the bed of affliction. By hope, I do not mean a dream that the affliction will disappear and all things will be as they once were. No, true hope is the confident expectation of something better to come. It is the assurance that whatever suffering we may experience, a better tomorrow lies ahead. Moreover, it is the confidence our suffering is not without purpose. Such hope keeps us from despairing or allowing our illness to define us. It enables us to persevere during trying circumstances.

I have found hope in one place: the Christian faith. My faith journey did not begin because of my ailments, though many would testify that the megaphone of physical affliction drove them to consider the claims of the carpenter from Nazareth. Rather, my journey began at the moment physical suffering ends—death. Not my own of course, but the death of two high school classmates shortly after graduation. One fell to his death while climbing Calvert Cliffs on the western shore of the Chesapeake Bay, while the other died from an aggressive form of leukemia. Their deaths shook me to the core. I had to face the reality that not only people the age of grandparents die. Truth be told, however, I was not ready for my own earthly departure. Death scared me beyond measure.

Most of us journey through life focused on the press of the immediate, with little reflection about the big questions often arising in our youngest days on this earth. What happens upon death? Is this life all there is? How did we come into being, and is there a purpose to our lives beyond personal gain? These are questions we should, but few do, consider persistently until answered. Indeed, once challenged with the reality of death's near grip, I concluded I could not really live until I was ready to die. If you cannot face the inevitable, how can you deal with the unknowns in life?

Over the ensuing years, I talked to individuals from a variety of faiths, as well as those who were antagonistic to the notion of faith. In college, I sat under the teaching of a communist sociologist, an aggressively foul-mouthed, anti-religionist social geographer, and a variety of scientists who believed our existence was due to mere chance. They expressed that our purpose for being was nothing more than a quest for the survival of the fittest. I found their worldviews to be unconvincing and insufficient to address the challenges of life. They also gave no strategy to face our greatest enemy—death.

During this period, my older brother married and moved out of our childhood home. This left me in possession of all four drawers of the dresser we had shared throughout our childhood. In the top drawer was the one item he left behind—a Bible given to him in the third grade by a stranger standing outside the school he attended. I don't know why I left it there. Perhaps my upbringing left me with enough respect for this holy book that I could not just throw it in the trash. The day came when I picked it up and started reading through its pages.

As I read the claims of the Nazarene by whom we mark our calendars, I concluded—as did C. S. Lewis in his classic, *Mere Christianity*—that this one named Jesus was either just as he claimed to be, the Son of God come to give himself for us, or else he was the most despicable deceiver who has ever tread his feet on this earth. I could no longer embrace the notion of this humble carpenter as just one of many wise men who have appeared through history. Good men do not make the remarkable claims he made unless they are true. Thus, I came to experience what he spoke to a Jewish leader about on a dark night in a garden. I was born anew…or really, reborn from above.

As that Oxford don C. S. Lewis so well described, I embrace the Christian faith for the same reason I embrace the reality of our sun. For not only do I see the sun and feel its presence, but also by it I see the world around me. In like manner, I believe in the person of Christ not only because I have experienced his presence in my own life and seen his impact on the lives of others, but also because the Christian faith enables me to make sense of the world around me like nothing else does—especially human suffering.

I recognize there are many who see the evil in this world as evidence of no God. I have read the accounts of some who experienced the horrors of the Holocaust who declare that the atrocities they lived through swept the notion of God from the realm of possibility. Surely, they assert, if there was a God, he could have created a world in which such evil would not occur. Yes, he could have—but experience tells us he did not. I cannot with honesty say how I would have responded to such horrors perpetrated by men against others had I walked through them. But is it proper to blame God for the evil of men? The inexplicable actions of men do not incline us to doubt their existence. Why should our inability to understand why God permits evil cause us to conclude he must not exist? Does the existence of

God depend on his acting the way *we* think he should? While there are some who have abandoned any vestige of faith in the face of horrible evil, many have also stood strong before such assaults and give testimony to faith's enabling power in their lives through such times.

Others struggle with the terror of natural disasters, either biological or geological. The seemingly arbitrary way physical affliction strikes individuals troubles the human heart. So much so, that some question whether a good God could have created a world in which such tragedies would befall its human inhabitants. In an era where most view the actions of men to have altered something as complex as our global climate, do we so quickly reject the notion that man himself has altered the original order of creation? Isn't it possible the physical world in which we dwell has been so altered by the evil of men that the ebb and flow of its actions are not as its Designer intended? Is it man or God who should be blamed for these natural terrors?

I firmly believe that how one views the reality of an afterlife will have a profound impact on the experience of chronic suffering. As stated multiple times in the preceding chapters, how you respond to physical suffering will ultimately determine whether you thrive in this life. If you believe suffering has no purpose apart from bringing misery, I do not know how you can fail to fall into despair. But if you believe even suffering has a purpose and hope exists beyond this life, you can face this and other challenges with resilience. There are marvelous examples of individuals who have done so and serve as encouragers for others.

Joni Eareckson Tada, mentioned in an earlier chapter, is one such example. She became a quadriplegic at a young age after a diving accident. By every account, her life is a beautiful fragrance to those blessed with knowing her. She has devoted her life to helping others experiencing substantial chronic suffering and is leaving the world a better place because of her life. Joni is a devout individual who embraces the Christian faith. She readily and joyfully declares that her faith empowers her to face her challenges with joy, as well as giving the confident assurance her suffering is not the final chapter of her story.

I opened this book by sharing my experience the day I learned there was no medical solution for the incessant back pain rendering my life nearly unbearable. As I sat in the car outside my university office, I wept like I have only once since this moment in my life—upon learning of my son's death. I did not think I could nor wanted to go on living with such intense unremitting pain. The darkness that descended on my life in this moment was emotionally shattering. Never before or since did I sense such personal despair. As the anguish permeated my being, I bore its weight . . . alone.

Fortunately, in the years preceding this moment I had spent many hours reading, meditating on, and teaching the Bible. As the storm of despair crashed into my life like so many waves on a shore, words from Scripture surfaced from the depth of my being. I remembered the character and promises of this one who had given his own son for me. In those darkest moments on the cross, the son expressed his own sense of abandonment. But as subsequent events showed, he was neither abandoned nor truly alone. I quickly came to the settled conviction that if this newest affliction was God's will for me, he would also provide the strength for me to bear it in a way that would honor him. In that moment, like the removal of a heavy physical weight, I could sense the burden of despair lifted from my being. I do not fear that those who know me best would contradict me when I write that I have not experienced even momentary despair since that troubled day, though additional life-altering ailments have entered my life. This is a measure of God's grace and not my resilience.

In his fascinating book *At Day's Close: Night in Times Past*, author A. Roger Ekirch describes how before the arrival of gas and electric lighting, men misinterpreted the sounds and the barely discernible sights of the night. The dawn's light brought a clarity that dispersed the dread of the unknown. As human achievement brought physical light to the night, we began to better understand the workings of the nocturnal world around us, and fear of the night mostly vanished.

In like manner, the one who proclaimed himself to be the "light of the world" can bring clarity, and an understanding of purpose, to the afflictions we experience in this life. Throughout his walk on this earth, he showed his deep compassion for the suffering of men and women. His healing touch and words

Acknowledgments

Deepest thanks go to my incredibly patient wife, Sue. She has journeyed with me through numerous chronic ailments with grace and tremendous helpfulness. Enduring endless conversations about this book, in addition to reading innumerable drafts, were an added burden. Her love has been steadfast through it all, and I unreservedly give her mine. The idea for writing this book actually arose from our daughter. I am grateful for her willingness to include part of her story. She has demonstrated uncommon grace in living with chronic pain.

Many have been kind to read parts or all of the manuscript that ultimately emerged as this book. Among these are Tom Berndt, Charles Hodges, Ed Langston, Kate Craig, and Priscilla Potter. My friend and professional colleague Bud Weiser took on the unenviable task of helping me not to offend those with a decent knowledge of grammar, syntax, etc. In addition, several patients living with various incurable illnesses have read parts or all of the manuscript and provided invaluable feedback. I preserve their anonymity here in respect of their right to control who knows that they are among the millions of silent sufferers. All of these individuals helped make this book better, but remaining shortcomings within are fully my responsibility. Unnamed are the innumerable patients whom I have encountered professionally or personally who expanded my understanding of living with chronic illness. I am very grateful to Purdue University for providing a sabbatical leave, enabling me to devote time and energy to writing.

Sandra Wendel deployed her expertise and experience as an editor to guide this novice author through the process of turning a manuscript into a book. I am grateful for her wisdom and patience. Christina Roth applied her amazing skill as a copyeditor to make this a readable text. Her attention to detail while keeping the big picture in view is nothing short of remarkable. Editors are artisans in the best sense of the word. My thanks also go to Jennifer Hartmann, who proved herself to be a highly skilled proofreader. I am also grateful to Cathi Stevenson and Gwen Gades, seasoned pros who provided the exterior and interior design for this book, respectively.

Finally, few things affected me more than watching my mother with an incurable disease deteriorate one organ at a time. She handled progressive physical deterioration with grace and humor. Moments from the final weeks of her life, demonstrating her continued resilience, are indelibly etched into my memory. My father's example of patient loving kindness to the end of her days may well be the greatest gift he has given to their children. I owe immeasurable thanks to both of them.

Notes

Chapter 1.

1. Job's declaration "I am allotted months of emptiness, and nights of misery are apportioned to me" is from Job 7:3, *The Holy Bible, English Standard Version.* ESV® Text Edition: 2016. Copyright © 2001 by Crossway Bibles, a publishing ministry of Good News Publisher.

2. The frequency of various diseases was obtained from the following national organization websites: Multiple Sclerosis Foundation (www.msfocus.org); National Fibromyalgia Association (www.fmaware. org); Parkinson's Foundation (www.parkinson. org); Crohn's and Colitis Foundation (www. crohnscolitisfoundation.org); Arthritis Foundation (www.arthritis.org); Disabled World (www. disabled-world.com/disability/types/invisible/

3. I recognize healthcare is provided by a wide variety of practitioners. Many patients with chronic

ailments are cared for by nurse practitioners,
physician assistants, clinical pharmacists, and
others. Nevertheless, those with complex diagnoses
are generally cared for in the realm of medical
specialists. Therefore, for simplicity, I make
most references to doctors/physicians. The same
principles discussed in this book apply to other
members of the healthcare team.

Chapter 2.

1. For a helpful discussion of the limits of the disease
   theory in medicine, see Eric J. Cassell, *The Nature
   of Suffering and the Goals of Medicine*, 2nd ed.
   (Oxford: Oxford University Press, 2004), 3–15.

2. An insightful presentation of medically unexplained
   symptoms is found in S. Hatcher and B. Arroll,
   "Assessment and Management of Medically
   Unexplained Symptoms," *British Medical Journal*
   336 (May 2008): 1124–28.

3. The frequency of medically unexplained symptoms
   in primary care practices in England was published
   as V. Aggarwal et al., "The Epidemiology of Chronic
   Syndromes That Are Frequently Unexplained:
   Do They Have Common Associated Factors?,"
   International Journal of Epidemiology 35 (April
   2006): 468–76.

4. Inherent problems with diagnostic codes is
   described in a provocative piece by J. A. Singer:
   "How Government Killed the Medical Profession,"

reproduced from the May 2013 issue of *Reason* at https://www.cato.org/publications/commentary/ how-government-killed-medical-profession.

5. The study showing emergence of neurodegenerative symptoms over two to five years was published as J. M. A. Wijnands et al., "Health-Care Use Before a First Demyelinating Event Suggestive of Multiple Sclerosis Prodrome: A Matched Cohort Study," *Lancet Neurology* 16 (June 2017): 445–51.

Chapter 3.

1. A rare disease is defined as a disorder occurring in less than 200,000 people. The number of people with a rare disorder is about 30 million. The assertion that this equates to circling the globe one and a half times is made in the National Organization for Rare Disorders Rare Disease Fact Sheet 2018, https://rarediseases.org/wp-content/uploads/2014/11/NRD-1008-RareInsights_v1.pdf.

2. The quote from Benjamin Franklin can be found in *Poor Richard's Almanack*, Poor Richard Improved, 1750, Rocket Edition by John Craft, 1999, 58.

3. For an example of a study showing quality of life of spouses and partners being poorer than that of patients, see J. Rees, C. O'Boyle, and R. MacDonagh, "Quality of Life: Impact of Chronic Illness on the Partner," *Journal of the Royal Society of Medicine* 94 (November 2001): 563–66.

4. The survey of patients with multiple sclerosis was published as 2017 MS in America Survey, https://multiplesclerosis.net/infographic/ms-in-america-2017/.

5. The report of the American Academy of Pediatrics on off-label drug use for rare diseases was published as Committee on Drugs, "Off-Label Use of Drugs in Children," *Pediatrics* 133 (March 2014): 563–67.

6. The paper describing conflicts of interest with patient advocacy groups was published as M. S. McCoy et al., "Conflicts of Interest for Patient-Advocacy Organizations," *New England Journal of Medicine* 376 (March 2017): 880–85.

7. The study showing drugs used off-label for an ailment may be more effective than approved drugs was published as A. Ladanie et al., "Off-Label Treatments Were Not Consistently Better or Worse Than Approved Drug Treatments in Randomized Trials," *Journal of Clinical Epidemiology* (November 2017), doi: 10.1016/j.jclinepi.2017.11.006.

8. A comprehensive review of published studies raising concerns about the content of dietary supplements was published as T. Rocha, J. S. Amaral, and M. B. P. P. Oliveira, "Adulteration of Dietary Supplements by the Illegal Addition of Synthetic Drugs: A Review," *Comprehensive Reviews in Food Science and Food Safety* 15 (January 2016): 43–62.

Chapter 4.

1. C. S. Lewis's book, *The Problem of Pain*, is one of the most compelling discussions about the suffering pain brings and the philosophical and theological dilemma such suffering presents.

2. The National Insitutes of Health estimates were provided in a press release on August 11, 2015, and may be found at www.nccih.nih.gov/news/press/08112015.

3. The >500-billion-dollar estimate comes from a study published as D. J. Gaskin and P. Richard, "The Economic Costs of Pain in the United States," *Journal of Pain* 13 (August 2012): 715-724.

4. For a helpful discussion of the mystery of chronic pain, see Scott Fishman and Lisa Berger, "The Mysteries of Chronic Pain," chap. 3 in *The War on Pain* (New York: HarperCollins, 2000), 51–67.

5. For a study showing the impact of anxiety on trigeminal neuralgia pain, see S. H. Mousavi et al., "Concomitant Depression and Anxiety Negatively Affect Pain Outcomes in Surgically Managed Young Patients with Trigeminal Neuralgia: Long-Term Clinical Outcome," *Surgical Neurology International* 7 (November 2016): 98.

6. Dr. Elliot Krane, Chief of Pain Management Service at Packard Children's Hospital at Stanford University, has given a concise description of how chronic pain differs in his TED Talk, which can be

viewed at https://ed.ted.com/lessons/the-mystery-of-chronic-pain-elliot-krane.

7. The study on distraction provoked changes in neuronal responses to pain was published as C. Sprenger et al., "Attention Modulates Spinal Cord Responses to Pain," *Current Biology* 22 (June 2012): 1019–22.

Chapter 6.

1. The discussion on preparing physicians for handling the tension of uncertainty was published as A. L. Simpkin and R. M. Schwartzstein, "Tolerating Uncertainty—The Next Medical Revolution?," *New England Journal of Medicine* 375 (November 2016): 1713–15.

2. An example of a study showing distress in women awaiting the results of a biopsy can be found in S. Lebel et al., "Waiting for a Breast Biopsy: Psychosocial Consequences and Coping Strategies," *Journal of Psychosomatic Research* 55 (May 2003): 437–43.

3. Evidence that delayed diagnosis may enable activation of coping mechanism was presented in K. Poole et al., "Psychological Distress Associated with Waiting for Results of Diagnostic Investigations for Breast Disease," *The Breast* 8 (December 1999): 334–38.

4. The study of the response in patients diagnosed with epilepsy is published as R. S. Fisher et al., "The Impact of Epilepsy from the Patient's Perspective. I.

Descriptions and Subjective Perceptions," *Epilepsy Research* 41 (August 2000): 39–51.

5. An in-depth treatment of sadness versus depression can be found in A. V. Horwitz and J. C. Wakefield, *The Loss of Sadness: How Psychiatry Transformed Normal Sorrow into Depressive Disorder* (Oxford: Oxford University Press, 2012), 15–16.

6. An example of a study showing distress in spouses and partners of those diagnosed with a degenerative disease can be found in K. Strickland, A. Worth, and C. Kennedy, "The Experiences of Support Persons of People Newly Diagnosed with Multiple Sclerosis: An Interpretative Phenomenological Study," *Journal of Advanced Nursing* 71 (December 2015): 2811–21.

Chapter 7.

1. The quote from Abraham Lincoln is found at https://www.goodreads.com/quotes/722599-if-i-am-killed-i-can-die-but-once-but.

Chapter 8.

1. Research into the impact of decisional conflict is published as M. M. Becerra-Perez et al., "More Primary Care Patients Regret Health Decisions If They Experienced Decisional Conflict in the Consultation: A Secondary Analysis of a Multicenter Descriptive Study," *BMC Family Practice* 17 (November 2016): 156.

2. For evidence of the role sociocultural factors play in patient decisions regarding treatment, see Y. K. Lee et al., "Exploring Patient Values in Medical Decision Making: A Qualitative Study," *PLoS One* 8 (November 2013): e80051.

3. The review of the role of decision tools in considering patient values for medical decisions was published as D. Stacey et al., "Decision Aids for People Facing Health Treatment or Screening Decisions," *Cochrane Database for Systematic Reviews* 4 (April 2017):CD001431.

4. A study evaluating patient preferences for medical decision-making is published as G. S. Chung et al., "Predictors of Hospitalized Patients' Preferences for Physician-Directed Medical Decision-Making," *Journal of Medical Ethics* 38 (February 2012): 77–82.

Chapter 9.

1. The quote from Solomon is from Proverbs 11:12. *Holy Bible, New International Version*®, NIV®. Copyright © 1973, 1978, 1984, 2011 by Biblica, Inc.® Used by permission. All rights reserved worldwide.

Chapter 10.

1. Research on the inconsistency of neurologists defining that a relapse had occurred in MS patients was published as C. H. Hawkes and G. Giovannoni, "The McDonald Criteria for Multiple

Sclerosis: Time for Clarification," *Multiple Sclerosis* 16 (May 2010): 566–75.

Chapter 11.

1. The commentary by Drs. Groopman and Hartzband was published as J. Groopman and P. Hartzband, "The Power of Regret," *New England Journal of Medicine* 377 (October 2017): 1507–09.

2. Research showing that patients who blame themselves for an injury-producing accident do not cope well was published as D. E. Sholomskas, J. M. Steil, and J. K. Plummer, "The Spinal Cord Injured Revisited: The Relationship Between Self-Blame, Other-Blame and Coping," *Journal of Applied Social Psychology* 20 (July 1990): 548–74.

3. Stress among physicians involved in serious errors is reported in A. D. Waterman et al., "The Emotional Impact of Medical Errors on Practicing Physicians in the United States and Canada," *The Joint Commission Journal on Quality and Patient Safety* 33 (August 2007): 467–76.

4. Insight into the self-blame experienced by some in response to self-help gurus is provided by B. Delaney, "Deepak Chopra's Healing Talk Appears to Empower but Self-Blame Is Not Far Behind," *Guardian*, August 4, 2016.

5. Self-blame and depression association was published as R. Zahn et al., "The Role of Self-

Blame and Worthlessness in the Psychopathology of Major Depressive Disorder," *Journal of Affective Disorders* 186 (November 2015): 337–41.

Chapter 12.

1. The quote from Job is found in Job 16:2, *The Holy Bible, English Standard Version*. ESV® Text Edition: 2016. Copyright © 2001 by Crossway Bibles, a publishing ministry of Good News Publishers.

2. For a helpful review of current findings on the health implications of loneliness, see J. E. Brody, "The Surprising Effects of Loneliness on Health," *New York Times*, December 11, 2017.